Research as Development

RESEARCH AS DEVELOPMENT

Biomedical Research, Ethics, and Collaboration in Sri Lanka

SALLA SARIOLA AND BOB SIMPSON

CORNELL UNIVERSITY PRESS
ITHACA AND LONDON

First published 2019 by Cornell University Press

Library of Congress Cataloging-in-Publication Data

Names: Sariola, Salla, author. | Simpson, Bob, 1956– author.
Title: Research as development : biomedical research, ethics, and
    collaboration in Sri Lanka / by Salla Sariola and Bob Simpson.
Description: Ithaca : Cornell University Press, 2019. | Includes
    bibliographical references and index.
Identifiers: LCCN 2018042027 (print) | LCCN 2018043945 (ebook) |
    ISBN 9781501733611 (e-book pdf) | ISBN 9781501733628
    (e-book epub/mobi) | ISBN 9781501733604 | ISBN
    9781501733604 (cloth)
Subjects: LCSH: Medicine—Research—Sri Lanka. | Medicine—
    Research—International cooperation. | Clinical trials—Moral and
    ethical aspects—Sri Lanka. | Medical ethics—Sri Lanka. | Bioethics—
    Sri Lanka. | Medical economics—Sri Lanka.
Classification: LCC R854.S72 (ebook) | LCC R854.S72 S37 2019 (print) |
    DDC 610.7205493—dc23
LC record available at https://lccn.loc.gov/2018042027

Contents

Acknowledgments

Collaboration is not an event but a process and, moreover, the relationships of which it is made unfold over many years. Consequently, the book we have written is shot through with the insights and efforts of many others to whom we are eternally grateful.

Our work in Sri Lanka was made possible by the generous and accommodating responses of many people. In particular we would like to thank colleagues associated with the South Asian Clinical Toxicology Research Collaboration (SACTRC) for the access we were given to their work conducting clinical trials and much more. We owe a particular debt of gratitude to Andrew Dawson, Michael Eddleston, Nick Buckley, Bishan Rajapakse, Mark Perera, and Melissa Pearson.

At the Colombo Medical Faculty we were given excellent assistance by Vajira Dissanayake, Rohan Jayasekera, Hemantha Senanayake, and many others.

We would also like to acknowledge the many other people who have shaped our understanding of the Sri Lankan research environment and, in particular, Sarath "Chubby" Arseculeratne, Arosha Dissanayake, Harshini Rajapakse, Athula Sumathipala, and Sisira Siribaddana.

Finally, our work in Sri Lanka would not have been possible were it not for the generosity and patience of the many doctors, nurses, administrators, clinical research assistants, and medical students who gave us their time in order to show us the world in which they lived and worked.

We would like to express a debt of gratitude to coresearchers on the International Science and Bioethics Collaborations project and specifically to Marilyn Strathern, who was the project's principal investigator; to Monica Konrad and Margaret Sleeboom-Faulkner, who were fellow coinvestigators; to Seyoung Hwang and Birgit Buergi, who were research associates; and to doctoral students Rachel Douglas-Jones and Achim Rosemann. The project was funded by the Economic and Social Research Council [no. RES-062-23-0215].

Ideas from the ISBC-project were carried forward and incubated in a subsequent project entitled Biomedical and Health Experimentation in South Asia. We are grateful to our collaborators on this project for the fertile environment they provided for us to develop our thinking and writing. In particular, we would like to thank Roger Jeffery (PI), Ian Harper, Amar Jesani, Vajira Dissanayake (Co-Is), Neha Madhiwalla, Anuj Kapilashrami, Jeevan Raj Sharma (collaborators), and research assistants Tharindi Udalagama, Deapica Ravindran, Anand Kumar, and Rekha Khatri.

As the writing of this book spans over a decade, numerous people have contributed to the thinking behind it. Salla would like to acknowledge the Ethox Centre, Nuffield Department of Population Health, University of Oxford, where she worked on a generous grant from the Wellcome Trust (Global Health Bioethics Network strategic award 096527). We are grateful that Bob was able to join Ethox as an academic visitor in 2014 so that we could work on the manuscript together. At Ethox, the writing benefitted hugely from conversations with Ruchi Baxi, Ariella Binik, Mikey Dunn, Ruth Horn, Maureen Kelley, Angeliki Kerasidou, Patricia Kingori, Mike Parker, and Mark Sheehan. Salla would also like to thank colleagues at the Global Health Bioethics Network: Susi Bull, Mary Chambers, Phaik Yeong Cheah, Nicola Desmond, Dorcas Kamuya, Elise van der Elst, Bernadette Kombo, Kevin Marsh, Vicki Marsh, Sassy Molyneux, Deborah Nyirenda, Lindsey Reynolds, and Eduard Sanders. Friends and colleagues in and around Oxford who were vital for thinking through this book also include

Alex Alvergne, Mwenza Blell, Tom Henfrey, Ann Kelly, akshay khanna, Catherine M. Montgomery, Matthäus Rest, and Olly Owen.

The present work has benefitted greatly from the advice, encouragement, and critique of colleagues in Durham University, Department of Anthropology, including Hannah Brown, Michael Carrithers, Dhana Hughes, Gina Porter, Andrew Russell, Maurice Said, Tom Widger, Tom Yarrow, and Peter Phillimore (University of Newcastle). Justin Dixon deserves a special mention for his assistance as a diligent and perceptive proofreader. Justin's contributions were crucial in getting the book into its final form.

Salla would like to acknowledge several colleagues in Finland for their inspiration and support: Sampsa Hyysalo, Mianna Meskus, Elina Oinas, Tiia Sudenkaarne, and Heta Tarkkala.

We are particularly grateful to the production team at Cornell University Press and to Jim Lance as senior editor for the efficient way in which the publication process has been handled. We would also like to thank the three anonymous reviewers whose comments have been enormously helpful.

Whilst contributions from all the above have gone into the writing of this book, responsibility for its final form is entirely our own.

Earlier versions of some sections of the book have been published elsewhere. We would like to thank Sage Publications for allowing us to reuse sections of Simpson, B., & Sariola, S. (2012), Blinding authority: Randomized clinical trials and the production of global scientific knowledge in contemporary Sri Lanka, *Science, Technology & Human Values*, 37(5), 555–575; Simpson, B. (2017), The 'we' in the me: A response to Prainsack, *Science, Technology & Human Values*, 43(1), 45–55; Oxford University Press for permission to reuse sections of Simpson, B. (2011), Capacity Building in Developing World Bioethics: Perspectives on Biomedicine and Biomedical Ethics in Contemporary Sri Lanka, from *Bioethics Around the Globe* edited by Catherine Myser; Elsevier for permission to reuse sections of Sariola, S., & Simpson, B. (2011), Theorising the "human subject" in biomedical research: International clinical trials and bioethics discourses in contemporary Sri Lanka, *Social Science and Medicine*, 73(4), 515–521; and Palgrave Journals for permission to reuse sections of Sariola, S., & Simpson, B. (2013), Precarious ethics: Toxicology research among self-poisoning hospital admissions in Sri Lanka, *BioSocieties*, 8(1), 41–57.

Research as Development

Chapter 1

International Collaborative Research in Biomedicine

A Form of Development?

On March 18, 2009, a workshop took place in the Faculty of Medicine of the University of Colombo in Sri Lanka. Under the watchful portraits of faculty deans and other eminent physicians extending back to colonial times, a group of some fifty doctors, ethicists, and social scientists came together to consider the ethics of international collaboration in biomedical research. The event took place against a backdrop of growing interest in the engagement of local researchers with international partners. Specifically it was concerned with the way that these engagements were taking shape in the form of internationally sponsored clinical trials.

The Colombo workshop occurred during the early stages of the ethnographic research on which this book is based. The International Science and Bioethics Collaboration (ISBC) project, of which we, the authors, were a part, had set out to study the complex entanglement of research, ethics, and collaboration with the broader questions of scientific and economic development.[1] Back in 2009 we were able to work with staff of the Faculty of Medicine of the University of Colombo (specifically the Human Genetics

Unit and the faculty's Ethics Review Committee) to organize the event. Furthermore, we were able to run it as a pre-congress workshop of the Sri Lanka Medical Association's 122nd Annual Scientific Sessions. This event proved to be a crucial introduction to the field of biomedical research, collaboration, and bioethics that we had set out to study.

The day began, as is customary, with an "inauguration." A panel comprising the president of the Sri Lanka Medical Association, the chair of the Ethics Committee of the Sri Lanka Medical Association, and both the chair of the Ethics Committee and the dean of the Colombo Faculty of Medicine gave their welcomes and good wishes to the assembled audience. The speeches were brief yet gave significant recognition and endorsement to the day's business. As if to capture yet further the gravitas of the place and the people assembled, certificates were given out to students who had recently qualified in an ethics course. The course, entitled "Ethical and Regulatory Aspects of Clinical Research," had been run by the Bioethics Department of the U.S. National Institutes of Health by remote link from Maryland. The linkage with the Annual Scientific Sessions and the presence of several key people from the world of ethics and medicine in Sri Lanka marked the event as one of considerable importance. A photographer was on hand to capture the assembled personnel in a group photograph.

The event was made to appear as a simple extension of custom and tradition, but the events of the day highlighted something more than that: a growing interest in and concern about ethics and international science collaboration. Among other things, the discussions that took place made it clear that the basic conceptual vocabulary of "research," "ethics," and "collaboration"—and the ends to which these are put—are far from stable. Rather they are fluid, contested, and contingent concepts. A primary aim of this book is to describe this conceptual instability in context so that we may understand just what is at stake for bioethics in the turbulence that is introduced when researchers collaborate in order to carry out clinical trials. Indeed, the engagement with foreign researchers and funding sources was no simple matter of importing research, ethics, and collaboration; rather, it resonated strongly with broader questions of culture, politics, and questions of development.

The Colombo workshop was the first of several that were held across Asia. They featured as part of our public engagement plans as specified in our original proposal to the project's funder, the United Kingdom's Economic and

Social Research Council. The workshops were an important opportunity for us to engage with the stakeholders who might be considered our end users— or, in more recent parlance, those on whom our research might have an impact. The workshops were in many respects a signal of our collaborative intent. As such, the Colombo event was extremely useful in establishing visibility for our research among Sri Lankan biomedical researchers, and it also provided us with insights into a very public form of reasoning: it was, so to speak, an exercise of the collective ethical imagination.

We were quickly drawn into the processes of interpretation, questioning, negotiation, and guesswork that go on behind and in response to the more categorical and authoritative assertions that are featured in the protocols and guidelines that govern the ethics of international collaborations. We had, without really realizing it at the time, set up what George Marcus (2000) has called a *para-site,* a participatory space in which a variety of discursive and interdisciplinary interactions can unfold. This particular para-site might be said to have successfully captured subjects in a reflective mode. Equally, however, it also captured ourselves as researchers as an object of their gaze. In this mutual subjectification, there were not two networks but one, which met around a common interest in the interface between science, ethics, and society.

Once the pleasantries were over, the chairman opened by directing us to the day's agenda. The title of the opening presentation from Bob Simpson raised a question: Why Should We Be Concerned about the Ethics of International Collaboration?[2] The presentation pointed out the current ubiquity of collaboration in biomedicine and the growing complexities that are inherent in relationships that span north-south divides, such as in relation to research funding, benefit-sharing, double-standards, differing standards, and the way that cultural differences are appropriated, factored into, or ignored in the ethical evaluation of research. This presentation was followed by a response from the chair of the ethics committee of the Colombo Medical Faculty, who made it extremely clear why there should be concern about the ethics of international collaboration. As chair of one of the busiest ethics committees in Sri Lanka, he described the committee and its members as carrying a heavy responsibility when it comes to deciding on the ethics of research that originates outside Sri Lanka but is conducted within. It was clear from his presentation that decisions made by the committee are not simply about the ethics of human subject research but entail complex judgments on issues ranging from the scientific validity of the research through to its potential social benefits (what these might look like and how much, or little, is acceptable). The simple model of a researcher performing research on a human subject that might result in harm or detriment is replaced with a much more complicated picture in which developing-world researchers themselves might fall prey to exploitation—and, indeed, find themselves doing the exploiting on behalf of others.

The difficulty effecting any simple framing of ethics in biomedical research in a setting such as Sri Lanka was illustrated rather starkly in a reflection on the dictionary definitions of the word "collaboration"[3] as presented by the chair of the Ethics Committee. He gave two readings of collaboration. In the first definition—"to work with others on a joint project"—collaboration is presented as unproblematic and in many respects a self-evident activity for people to do. As such, it sits comfortably with the ubiquitous language of partnership, participation, multidisciplinary and interdisciplinary teams, and the hoped-for synergies that these engagements will bring. Drawing on multiple perspectives in a flat, nonhierarchical way is believed to offer a promise of added value; collaboration brings more robust knowledge, better solutions to existing problems, and deeper insights into future ones, with a heightened impetus to form positive, productive, and effective relationships (Nowotny, Scott, and Gibbons 2001; Strathern 2005, 2012). This was the first meaning of collaboration presented to the group, which conveyed what we might think of as the warm themes of collaboration.

However, as the chair's second definition made clear, the word *collaboration* also has its cooler themes: "to cooperate as a traitor, especially with an enemy occupying one's own country." This inflection of collaboration was broached at several points during the meeting as the participants reflected on the negative reciprocity that collaboration might entail. This is hardly surprising given that international collaborations often take place across major differentials of power, knowledge, and resources. Working across such differentials ushers in the possibility that collaboration will result in extraction and exploitation. Thus, although the positive desire for engagement with global research networks and institutions is widely in evidence, it is also the case that such collaborations invite anxieties and concerns about the motives of foreign researchers. These anxieties are easily transferred to the local researchers who work with them. In this reading, collaboration rouses suspicions of traitorous collusion with an enemy oppressor and a rejection of expected morals and values in the process.

The chair of the Colombo Medical Faculty's Ethics Committee put before the audience images depicting the fate of those who worked for the Nazis in France during World War II. To a backdrop of pictures of "collaborators"—stripped, with shaven heads—he expressed concerns that he and his colleagues could find themselves cast as this kind of collaborator. He spoke of the pressures of "getting things right" and the risk of public vilification should they approve, albeit in good faith, international projects that others see as ethically flawed.

The choice of visual references from World War II is an illustration of collaboration in its problematic forms, but it is revealing at another level as well. It is a poignant reminder of the way that fascism in Europe was also the source of other important genealogies of images and ideas. Of relevance here are the Nuremberg trials, in which Nazi doctors were prosecuted for medical research abuses committed in concentration camps. Out of these trials came the regulatory guidelines for ethical research that became known as the Declaration of Helsinki, which subsequently became the foundational charter of contemporary bioethics. Significantly, the genealogy of bioethics chosen by the chair of the Ethics Committee had been generated in Europe rather than closer to home. Indeed, what our preliminary workshop made abundantly clear was that, when it comes to the ethics of international collaboration in research, there are rhetorical moves that set out distinctions regarding what should and should not be incorporated locally when it comes to practices and values. In short, outlines were being drawn of what a "Sri Lankan research culture" might be, and, more importantly, what it should not be.

In the politeness afforded by abstraction, everybody at the workshop seemed to agree on the problem: unethical research practices. Conversations were mostly amicable and aimed at consensus. Yet there were also points at which tensions surfaced. How should the unethical be recognized? When international clinical trials are performed, *why* are they performed, *by whom, how,* and *to what ends?* In the debates that followed the chair's contribution, we had a glimpse of the local critiques of international collaboration. Allegations were made concerning complicity with foreign researchers, corrupt practices were intimated, and suggestions were made that some researchers were not acting in the nation's interest. In these discussions, a densely textured relationship between biomedical research, international collaboration, and bioethics began to unfold.

Although there was considerable enthusiasm for the ways in which "Western" research is framed and governed, anxieties were evident about the consequences of this approach for the development of an acceptably "Sri Lankan research culture" and how this fits with the nation and its future development. In these discussions, it became apparent that there were multiple versions of what that culture should be and how international collaboration should work in realizing it.

Research as Development: A Novel Entanglement?

Biomedical research and development are usually thought of as distinct and sequential. That is, we tend to think of research *and* development (as in "R&D") of a product or technology. The relationship is seen as linear, sequential, and inexorably future oriented. This configuration is made possible when there is the infrastructure, resources, and personnel to realize the relationship, as is often the case in societies that are economically and technologically advanced. By contrast, in societies that are resource-poor, the relationship between research and development is far from linear. Development efforts first have to create the conditions for research in order for future development to take place. Consistent with the practices of those with whom we worked, we look at this tangled relationship in practice—that is, biomedical research *as* development—or at least as an increasingly important piece of the complex mosaic of resources and relationships that are brought under the label of development.

We focus on the significant crossovers between research as systematic knowledge creation and innovation, and development as the orchestration of economic, material, and human resources to achieve growth, improvements in well-being, and sustainability as these are currently organized against a backdrop of globalization and the spread of neoliberal regimes of practice and value. The loci of our interest in research as development are the ways in which researchers set up international collaborations and particularly clinical trials, which typically bring together researchers to work across significant differentials of power and resources. A focus on these collaborations makes explicit the interests of those conducting the trials. As we go on to show, their aspirations extend beyond the specifics of scientific interest in a research question and play out into broader concerns. Participating in international collaborations as far as development is concerned is to engage in activities that will translate into economic and social benefits—a hoped-for future in which things will be better for individuals, institutions, and the nation (see Douglas-Jones and Shaffner 2017, particularly Boulding 2017; Ellison 2017; Hewlett 2017; LaHatte 2017). Powerful drivers of this activity are the proximal and longer-term increases in human capacity (jobs, training, management expertise, organizational skills, governance, and career development and qualifications) as well as material and infrastructural development (grants, buildings, information technology equipment, and laboratories).

Our interest in clinical trials as a vehicle for this kind of development in Sri Lanka takes place at a time when, as in many other countries, state-provided health care services are becoming increasingly decentralized, privatized, and more porous when it comes to outside intervention. Multi-site trials have been identified as a further symptom of this global drift toward neoliberal policies in health care provision in that they bring a growing entanglement of research experimentation with health care provision (for example, see Petryna 2009). Under these circumstances, internationally sponsored clinical trialing finds fertile ground for growth. Engagement in international collaborations, whether with commercial pharmaceutical companies or public sector organizations such as universities and international nongovernmental organizations (NGOs), is seen as critical for improving this position. A global political and economic agenda that currently emphasizes open borders for intellectual property, and economies of knowledge and research activity, suggests the possibility of new forms of inclusivity. Under such circumstances, the relationship between research and development begins to take on some novel forms as economically developing nations configure their science policies within global health inequities, on the one hand (Kelly and Beisel 2011; Leach, Scoones, and Wynne 2005), and with an emerging "post-colonial technoscience" on the other (Abraham 2006; Anderson 2002, 2009; Harding 2008; Prasad 2006, 2009, 2014). Our work shows how local researchers forge collaborations and how research operates as both a tool and a target for development.

It may seem odd to be focusing on development at a time when much effort has gone into dissolving it as a coherent and meaningful category

(Yarrow and Venkatesan 2012, 7). Mindful of this observation, the point we wish to emphasize at the outset is an ethnographic one rather than an analytical one. Development, and the many forms this is thought to take, was an idea that the doctors, researchers, and clinicians with whom we worked were keen to link with the practice of biomedical research. International collaboration was seen as an important way to achieve its *telos:* a different future and the practical steps needed to achieve change toward it. Our interlocutors were keenly aware of the role that biomedicine and the research on which it relies could play in moving the nation forward. Thus, in our account, development is not a faceless diffusion but an active hope and desire carried forward by real people, whom we came to know well. As such we have tried to capture the workings of what Pieter De Vries has described as "the desiring machine," which "functions through the constitution of this lack (of knowledge, social capital, resources, etc.), which as a void gives body to all sorts of fads, theories and rationalisations" (De Vries 2007; see also Deleuze and Guattari 1987; Ferguson 1994). We, as researchers, were drawn into a loop in which those who might be presumed to be the target of development were in fact themselves drawing on the categories of development discourse to engage recursively, pragmatically, and creatively with it (Bruun Jensen and Winthereik 2013). They were using collaboration and clinical trials to gain the desired outcome of future development.

This process is no simple one-way, hegemonic flow that sees knowledge and technology flowing from the global north to the south, and resources flowing in the opposite direction. At the point where local actors enter into the global epistemes of biomedical science, we began to identify a radical deterritorialization in which the usual reference points of state, capital, individual enterprise, biomedical science, and development were being brought together in novel reconfigurations. Here we encountered uncertainty about what the problems of collaborations are and what is at stake. These questions were of great significance during the economic and political turmoil in which Sri Lanka found itself during the period of our fieldwork and not least as a result of the vicious and protracted civil war that raged in the background throughout. In our attempts to capture the fine grain of these encounters, the reflexive intentions of those who are the agents of development practice are central (Mosse 2005, 5–6).

In showing that, in the Sri Lankan case, the impetus for collaboration emerged from within the country rather than being driven solely by external interests, our work draws attention to the very particular dynamics that prevail in Sri Lanka. The specificity is important. For example, in her account of the development of human immunodeficiency virus (HIV) research in Uganda, Johanna Crane documented the "scrambling" to create research opportunities to carry out biomedical research in Africa (Crane 2013,16). She describes how U.S. interests in developing global health collaborations in Uganda led local doctors to respond with a mixture of gratitude and resentment. The gratitude came from the influx of resources; the resentment came from the power differentials that created a sense of exclusion. By contrast, the Sri Lankan researchers we describe here were proactive in their efforts to attract and embed international research in the country by means of sustainable international collaborations. Our focus here thus opens up novel perspectives on collaboration in that it brings to the fore the practice of research. Unlike other studies of international research, it reveals how researchers operate pragmatically and strategically to accomplish collaboration on their terms and in ways that work in their own setting.

By focusing on the activities of researchers locally, we leave behind many of the dichotomies with which the literature on development and clinical trials is strewn. In particular, we address a common analytical blind spot regarding the diffusion of knowledge and the conceptual underpinnings in some of the empirical studies of science. Amit Prasad, for example, argues that these approaches "rarely analyze the construction of the west versus non-west techno-cultural divide, which undergirds diffusion models and has an impact not just on analyses of scientific research and policy formulations but also on ideological and discursive construction of non-western cultures as inferior and non-creative" (2006, 221). These binaries divide the West from the rest, the developed from the developing, the global north from the global south, and the West from the East. In this view, the binary draws attention to the deficits that lie on one of its sides. Knowledge, power, and resources are assumed to be all out of kilter, and it is the object of those who control the levers of international development to rebalance them if progress and improvement are to be achieved. Their objective is typically seen as being hampered by poor infrastructure, maldistribution of resources, and corruption and poor governance in the target nations of development interventions.

The relationship that emerges under these conditions is reminiscent of what we call the hub-and-spoke model, with developing countries ranged around the rim and the flow of resources, mostly in the form of "aid," moving outward from a resource-rich center. The centralized distribution of resources along the spokes is assumed to bring progress around the rim. Progress is generally seen in terms of the degree to which the techno-rational systems of the West are imitated at the periphery—and here we would include the growing imbrication of biomedical science and bioethics. In the context of biomedical research and international collaboration explored here, the hub-and-spoke model identifies partners in northern universities and industries with local partners and concentrates on the latter acquiring the procedures and practices of the former. It is assumed in this model that northern partners bring expertise not available locally, and research is heavily inflected with the notion of "capacity building," which for some northern researchers of global health becomes something of an ethical obligation (Beran et al. 2017). In this model, the periphery is marked by deficit when it comes to science, technology, and bioethics, with the creation and transfer of new knowledge and wealth typically being framed by policy-makers in the north rather than by those in the south. As Mark Duffield argues, this conceptualization results in ideological legitimations of the drive to control: "the borderlands are . . . imagined spaces of breakdown, excess and want that exist in and through a reforming urge to govern, that is, to reorder the relationship between people and things, including ourselves, to achieve desired outcomes" (2002, 1053). Bagele Chilisa (2005), in an illuminating account of HIV/AIDS educational research in Botswana, showed how collaborative research between low- and high-income countries tends to fall into this mold. Chilisa argued that failing to engage with local knowledge systems is symptomatic of this thinking and a colonial throwback in which "the colonized were regarded as empty vessels to be filled" (2005, 676).

Randomized Controlled Trials: Beyond Empty Vessels

Belying the image of the "empty vessel" is a rather more complex engagement between scientific research and development. Harry M. Marks has attributed the establishment and rapid growth of clinical trials in the last quarter of the nineteenth century and early twentieth century to the emergence of what he refers to as "rational therapeutics"—that is, treatments that are based on proven efficacy rather than the marketing hubris of the late nineteenth century and early part of the twentieth (1997, 17–41). At that time, U.S. and European markets displayed an abundance of remedies and potions that were sold by manufacturers and other commercial entities with little by way of evidence of efficacy. Marks argued that some of these products were mere placebos; some were no more than concoctions of dye, sugar, alcohol, or codeine, yet all were marketed vigorously with colorful advertisements as cures for all ills (Marks 1997, 19). The medical fraternity, with the American Medical Association's Council on Pharmacy and Chemistry in the vanguard, felt that leaving the commercial distribution of medicines unchecked would taint the efforts then under way to consolidate the power and influence of the medical profession.

A solution was needed that would distinguish the legitimate from the bogus claims as to the efficacy of drugs, while at the same time locating prescription knowledge and practices within the professions rather than in the commercial realms where lay- or self-prescription were the norm. Such moves would ensure the reputation and power of the medical profession in the face of commercial activities beyond its control. Moreover, developments in laboratory techniques and computation have provided ever new ways to come up with evidence of what does and does not work. "A rational, as opposed to an empirical [here: observed by the physician or patient] remedy, was one whose effects were demonstrable in the laboratory and ideally acted on the cause, not on the symptoms, of disease" (Marks 1997, 21).

In the period after World War II, major developments in identifying the efficacy of antibiotics and steroids coupled with advances in statistical methods to handle big data sets created the conditions for large-scale experimentation. The method set in place by public health statistician Bradford Hill (1990) involved randomization, investigators blinded to interventions, and predefined end points and sample sizes for validity. These techniques were consolidated into what is now recognized as the widely adopted randomized controlled trial (RCT). The first RCT, which trialed the antibiotic streptomycin for tuberculosis (TB), was officially carried out in the United Kingdom by the Medical Research Council (MRC) between 1946 and 1948 (MRC 1948). The subjects were allocated into different treatment groups under carefully monitored conditions so that the effects and efficacy might be evaluated (Timmermans and Berg 2003).

Often the story of RCTs has been reported in ways that suggest that their methodological development is a Western one or, conversely, that RCTs are new arrivals in countries beyond Europe and the United States. However, we draw attention to some of the trials that have taken place in non-Western countries that, although of lesser visibility, are nonetheless an important part of the history of clinical trials, evidence-based medicine, and the governance of RCTs internationally. These trials constitute an important detail in our argument for alternatives to the hub-and-spoke model in which countries in the global south are seen as mere recipients of international research activity. The history of clinical trials is also one in which the field of bioethics is implicated, because controversies over trial practices were usually followed by a tightening of ethics regulation.

Melissa Graboyes's (2014, 2015) work on human experimentation in Africa shows that the history of medicine is deficient in its understanding of the role played by the research that went into various diseases in the colonies. After World War II, extensive clinical research on sleeping sickness, malaria, leprosy, river blindness, and elephantiasis was taking place in East Africa (Graboyes 2014, 2015), while smallpox and kala-azar (visceral leishmaniasis) were studied in India (Bhattacharya 2006; Dutta 2008), and leprosy and TB in Nigeria (Manton 2011). These studies drew in hundreds of thousands of people for whom therapy was mixed with experimentation. Graboyes (2014) has argued that research in Africa was by no means exceptional in the ways in which people were "recruited." Across many regions, people found themselves involved in trials, especially those living in confined settings or who otherwise lacked access to health care. Often they had been misinformed about the nature of the research, and they were, in some instances, enrolled under duress (Graboyes 2014, 380). Highlighting this particular dynamic in the history of medicine in the colonies as a circulating one, rather than a one-way, hub-and-spoke type of diffusion, has important consequences:

> By substituting 'project' with 'process' as the object of study, the whole perspective of examining the history of medicine changes. While for the former the modernity–tradition dichotomy is a requisite of analysis, in the latter the clear-cut dichotomy or opposition between modern and traditional and non-Western medicines becomes irrelevant due to their interaction, accommodation and co-ordination, although spasmodic and marked by instances of resistance and conflict, within the framework of reconstruction of modern medicine. (Ebrahimnejad 2009, 25)

In the post-war era, Jill Fisher has argued, there was a sense in the United States that American doctors were above the conduct of ethically questionable research and that the events in Nazi Germany were an exception rather than the norm (2009, 20). This assumption was brought into question by the Tuskegee experiment conducted between 1932 and 1974, in which African Americans, mostly poor sharecroppers, were recruited into a study of the natural history of syphilis. The scandal broke when it emerged that the volunteers were not treated for their condition despite the discovery, partway through the study, that antibiotics could cure syphilis. The furor over this experiment led to new guidelines for the conduct of RCTs and tighter ethics guidelines to ensure the protection of the participants (National Commission for the Protection of Human Subjects 1978). The same group of researchers were later implicated in another morally questionable trial that they conducted after World War II. Between 1947 and 1948 in Guatemala—which was then under U.S. protection—the researchers infected prisoners, psychiatric patients in asylums, and orphans in institutions with gonorrhoea and syphilis in order to follow the development of the disease and with a view to testing different medicines. This trial did not receive public attention until 2010, when the U.S. government officially apologized to those affected by the experiments (Löwy 2011).

The study in Guatemala was not unique in the way in which it recruited populations. Until the 1960s, the majority of trials in the United States were conducted on prison populations, soldiers, and people in mental health institutions (Cooper and Waldby 2014, 146; Fisher 2009, 20–23). In 1962, legislative changes in the United States placed restrictions on this form of trialing. Trial phases were introduced, and restrictions were put in place regarding the inclusion of incarcerated and institutionalized populations (Cooper and Waldby 2014, 132). The shifting regulatory landscape in the United States created a need to look for experimental populations more widely (Petryna 2005, 2009; Sunder Rajan 2005b, 2006).

The immutability and increasing mobility of the trials apparatus was consolidated on a global scale through ever more scrupulous adherence to rules and procedures for the conduct of trials. A key document in this regard was the International Council for Harmonization Good Clinical Practice Guidelines (ICH-GCP), produced in the mid-1990s (Abraham and Reed 2002). These guidelines were meant to ensure that commercial research was conducted to the same standards irrespective of location. Evidence that these guidelines have been followed faithfully guarantees the recognition and acceptance of the results by wider scientific publics, including drug regulatory bodies, academic peers, and journal audiences. Crucially, however, the demonstrable capacity to index local practice to "global standards" is for the consideration of national bodies such as the U.S. Food and Drug Administration (FDA), which grant licenses for new pharmaceutical products to enter lucrative international markets.

Predictably, this in turn has led to concerns about the ways in which variation in the interpretation and application of guidelines in different jurisdictions can have variable consequences. For instance, Adriana Petryna described a case in which a drug was released for general use in Nigeria while still being trialed in the United States. The resulting controversy led to the first global lawsuit against a drug company (2009, 39). Another example comes from a commercial pre-exposure HIV prophylaxis (PreP) study conducted in 2004 by Gilead in Cambodia, Cameroon, Malawi, Nigeria, and Thailand. This trial was called off midway because of resistance by local sex workers and LGBT activists (Cooper 2013; Singh and Mills 2005; Ukpong and Peterson 2009). The participating communities were critical of the fact that their needs and demands for post-trial access were not included in the protocol. Cases like this have led to organizations such as the Council for International Organizations of Medical Sciences (CIOMS) demanding the incorporation of community engagement as an ethical expectation for all medical research.

In summary, trials have been conducted in non-Euro-American locations since the inception of the RCT methodology. This observation suggests important circularities as the knowledge generated by the experiments carried out at the peripheries is brought back to Europe and America. These circularities are also paralleled by global developments in ethics regulation after controversies that have unfolded during these experiments. These are important examples that contextualize the arguments we develop here; they problematize the assumption that knowledge and expertise only flow in one global direction, north to south. They also bring into view the active role that local researchers have played in shaping research activity.

Yet the problems described in these examples do not augur well for collaboration's warm themes—that is, the formation of equitable and complementary relationships as the basis of international research. The dominant relationship appears to be one in which local natural and human resources are plundered under the auspices of development while control is maintained by the institutions of the global north, a view that resonates with the ethics chair's uncomfortable allusion to the cooler themes inherent in research collaboration. Scholars such as Sheila Jasanoff (2014), Sandra Harding (2008), Itty Abraham (2006), and Susantha Goonatilake (1998) have highlighted these power inequalities. The field of scientific practice is not a level one when it comes to knowledge creation and transfer. Their works suggest that the terms and conditions under which experimental research is conducted have already been established for economically developed countries, and the less economically developed ones then have little chance to influence what has gone on farther up the chain of knowledge creation and transfer.

In this regard, Arjun Appadurai has drawn attention to an epistemological exclusion that operates around the production and validation of knowledge, particularly as it relates to the medical sciences (2000, 2). The rapid movement of people, capital, information, and resources around the globe makes it difficult for many nations to map out the forms and meanings of this knowledge on their own terms. The result is a systematic marginalization from setting new agendas for technological innovation and scientific research. To date, the main targets for this critique have been agreements around patenting, copyright, and ownership. Instigated by the leading industrial countries, trade sanctions have become closely linked to infringements of intellectual property rights through the World Trade Organization's 1994 General Agreement on Tariffs and Trade. Eventually consolidated into TRIPS (Trade Related Aspects of Intellectual Property Rights Including Counterfeit Goods), such agreements made it possible to appropriate things that previously could never have been imagined as property: seeds, bacteria, Ayurvedic treatments, traditional agricultural practices, artistic designs, and so on. After protest about the damaging effect this agreement was having on many developing world countries, the original TRIPS agreement was modified in 2001 to allow signatories to protect public health by ensuring access to pharmaceuticals and differential patenting arrangements for some drugs. The drift toward epistemological exclusion, however, remains pronounced in high-technology fields such as genomics and pharmaceutical testing in which value lies primarily in globally transferable databases.

The importance of these power discrepancies between the global north and south and their implications for knowledge production are serious; however, as we go on to illustrate, this is not the whole story. Indeed, by considering the relationship between clinical trials, bioethics, and collaboration in practice, we hope to extend the story in important ways (and for an example of a similar endeavor in pharmaceutical development in South Africa, see Pollock 2014). In the account we present, three factors are seen to mark out this relationship as one that confounds the normative assumptions arising from a hub-and-spoke model.

First, as participants at the collaboration workshop we described earlier demonstrate, we are dealing with experts and expert systems for which there can be mutual and comparable levels of competence between practitioners from the global north and south. Indeed, not only were many of the "local" practitioners we worked with Western trained, several were also expatriate Sri Lankans who had returned to the island "as if" they were from the global north, and who were able to activate local networks based on familiarity and trust (see chapter 4). In other words, there is no simple gradient flowing from north to south but a rather more complex history of migration back and forth on which contemporary collaborations are often built.

Second, unlike the material resources and commodities that animate much of the development critique, we are here dealing primarily with knowledge and its inherent potentiality to create different futures. As Karen-Sue Taussig, Klaus Hoeyer, and Stefan Helmreich put it in their exploration of the concept of potential, "in biomedical practices, potentiality indexes a gap between what is and what might, could, or even should be" (2013, S5). In short, when talking about knowledge in the context of research and development, we are dealing with a very particular kind of resource. It is one that is not so easily governed by the mechanisms that are conventionally used to create scarcity, drive up value and cost, and achieve the kinds of accumulation on which global capitalism is mostly built. Indeed, one of the central themes running throughout the book is that collaboration, at least in theory, begins with the presumption of freely shared knowledge, ideas, and discoveries as the key to progress and betterment (see chapter 5). The idea of potential becomes a key driver of hope and expectation. It would no doubt be naïve to assume a perfect freedom in operation when people describe what they are doing as "collaboration"; nonetheless, in the contexts discussed here we would argue that there is an attempt to signal a different relationship from that which figures in the hub-and-spoke model. There is an attempt to achieve a different kind of positionality, power, and purchase among those working in and on behalf of developing world constituencies. A factor that aids this endeavor is the sheer velocity and replicability of information.

Here we arrive at our third distinguishing feature. The availability of information and communication technologies, although still far from even across the global north-south divide, does enable local doctors, clinicians, and researchers to participate in global knowledge systems directly. Although spatially far apart, a trial conducted in Sri Lanka is easily articulated by means of the wormholes of the worldwide web to the laboratory benches and data sets of richer countries. Collaboration in research might connect a bedside in rural Sri Lanka with the headquarters of a pharmaceutical headquarters in the United States or Australia. Samples and data might flow between laboratories and offices operating in different continents with human, economic, and intellectual resources having to be managed at every stage (see chapter 3).

An ethnographic approach to these issues shifts the focus from biomedical and technological innovation per se onto power relations and practices played out in day-to-day social relations. Our ethnographic exploration of research as development might thus be seen as an exercise in giving voice. However, as we go on to show, this is not the voice of the oppressed, muted, and downtrodden but that of various professionals and experts who in their work seek to negotiate with global knowledge systems to achieve a range of desired outcomes.

Assemblages and Rhizomes

A model that gets us closer to understanding these relationships is provided by Aihwa Ong and Stephen Collier's (2005) idea of the "global assemblage." The idea of an assemblage is drawn from a conceptual vocabulary that originates in the work of Gilles Deleuze and Félix Guattari (1987) and their efforts to arrive at new ways of writing and thinking about culture and mental life. The French term that is typically translated into English as assemblage is *agencement*, meaning "an arrangement," as in the parts of a machine or body. Rendered into English, the idea of an assemblage gives the sense of more actively bringing things together, as in a collage (Phillips 2006). *Global assemblage*, as used here, refers to projects of various kinds that have global reach and are refracted through particular localities as scaled and structured versions of dominant models and paradigms.

Although the notion of concepts, ideas, and discourses that travel is not inherently new, what is helpful in Ong and Collier's formulation is the ability to manage the scales at work when this happens When dealing with networks that operate across multiple sites in the process of globalization, the idea of the assemblage brings into view the way that international policies, acts, ratifications, and standards come to operate in widely differing contexts. It also makes visible the power relations inherent in shifts of scale. Studying such forms thus offers a methodological *entré* into what are otherwise vague conceptualizations of the notion of globalization. Examples of these forms gathered by Ong and Collier include HIV prevention, ideas of human rights, banking, and the regulation of food production. All these examples reveal ideas and practices that easily transgress territories and boundaries and are readily fluid and scalable across regions, nations, and cultures.

To think of biomedical research, bioethics, research governance, the operation of clinical trials, and the very idea of collaboration itself as parts of an assemblage is to bring into question the presumptions of a hub-and-spoke model by drawing closer attention to the active role that those on the "periphery" play in shaping these notions. Furthermore, they do not just receive ready-made conceptual packages but make these in practice, thereby creating scientific discourses that are shot through with local expressions of society and culture (see chapter 6).

The second notion we introduce to understand the ways in which international collaborations operate is that of the *rhizome*, which is helpful in trying to understand the seemingly random connections that make up an international collaboration (Douglas-Jones and Sariola 2009). As Timothy K. Choy and colleagues suggest, the rhizome "offers a way to talk about fields and lines of connecting, relating, interpenetrating, becoming, and transforming. One point is crucial: The rhizome not only refuses arborescent being but it also requires a nonarborescent analysis. Its organization—and the proper organization of thought—is emergent through the actualization of connections" (2009, 384). The relevance of this imagery to our work is that it pulls us even further away from the hub-and-spoke model of collaborative relations and opens these up as a field of possibilities in which connections are being continually and creatively made and un-made.

As with the rhizome as it occurs in the natural world, the system of growth and propagation of collaborations—in which we will necessarily include our-selves—is one that is irregular and continuous, with connections liable to form between any points in the network. The analogy is helpful when it comes to providing an account of exactly what happens when a collabora-tion is established. At one level what happens is formal, technical, and pro-cedural, involving networks of professionals who occupy designated roles and statuses which may interact in impersonal ways. Yet it also engages a pro-foundly socialized vision of collaboration in which trust, respect, friendship, and camaraderie are valued and aspired to. Seeing this complex amalgam as rhizomatic rather than fixed and programmatic enables us to cut through the optimism in some development paradigms as well as the negativity with which this is greeted by critical commentators.

An Anthropology of Clinical Trials and Bioethics

In focusing on the entanglement of biomedical research, bioethics and de-velopment our work sits within a growing field of enquiry into scientific prac-tices in the global south (Biruk 2012; Brives 2013; Dixon 2017; Geissler and Molyneux 2011; Lairumbi et al. 2012; Le Marcis 2015; Montgomery 2015; Whyte 2011). Literature from Africa describes specifically how international research collaborations operate in the field, with attention paid to trial par-ticipants and their recruitment by local field staff (Brown and Green 2015; Dixon 2017; Kamuya et al. 2013; Kamuya et al. 2014; Kingori 2013; Kingori and Gerrets 2016; Molyneux et al. 2013; Sambakunsi et al. 2015). Another strong focus in this literature is the way in which clinical trials also create health care infrastructures that enable patients to access care they might not otherwise get (Crane 2013; Kingori 2015; Lairumbi et al. 2012; Petty and Heimer 2011; for a similar argument in relation to Russia, see Zvonareva et al. 2015). Historical aspects of public health organizations illuminate how colonial medical administrators were driven by an ethos of progress, enlightenment, and development and were preoccupied with medicine as part of an overall project of modernization—a legacy that still echoes in the rhetoric of many global health researchers today (Geissler and Molyneux 2011, 4).

These evident and obvious consequences of international research collab-oration we take to be first order—that is, having immediate and tangible effects on resources and health systems at the local level. An exploration of these effects runs through our account of research as development, but we also wish to throw light on a second order of consequences. Specifically, we explore a conceptual shift that is not always apparent in the accounts of development of the first order. It is a form of *epistemic* development that enables local players—doctors, clinicians, scientists, technicians, and other research staff in Sri Lanka—to participate, gain credibility, and indeed compete in the game of global scientific research (see chapters 5 and 6). Ethnographic interest, here, settles on the day-to-day running of clinical trials and the alterations carried out by researchers who are keen to align their practices and values with global systems of governance and regulation. Without these activities, such trials would not be workable in local settings.

Central to the achievement of workability is a concern to engage with bioethics as a primary source of values and concepts informing ethical research practice. This engagement is one of the key second order developments that we present in this book. As a varied and multifaceted discipline, bioethics emerged out of the encounter between advances in Western biomedicine and technology, and the Euro-American value systems in which these were situated (Jonsen 1998; see Campbell 2000 for critique of this unified narrative). In recent decades, bioethics has undergone considerable consolidation as a field of scholarship and expertise, a discipline, a profession, and an ideology. Its practitioners engage with questions of governance, law, economics, and philosophy in an effort to inform society as to how best to respond to the dilemmas that scientific advance presents—or, as is more often the case, appears to leave in its wake. Increasingly, these questions are not just ones that perturb those living in the global north, but with the global biomedical and technological advances bioethics itself has become a global project (Benatar 2002; Benatar, Daar, and Singer 2005; Hyder and Wali 2006; Myser 2011; Wahlberg et al. 2013).

Often in the guise of "capacity building," the growth of bioethics has brought about an alignment of local practices and concerns with those found in the global north (see, e.g., Simpson 2012; Douglas-Jones 2017). In low-income settings, this activity is interpreted in one of two ways. On the one hand, it is thought to protect the interests of nations and participants in the research encounters. Structures are put in place to ensure that research is carried out in socially and culturally relevant ways: communicating and eliciting informed consent along with other practices intended to ground the ethical credentials of research (Gikonyo et al. 2008; Molyneux et al. 2005b); establishing trust between communities (Gikonyo et al. 2008; Molyneux et al. 2005a); setting up ethics committees/institutional review boards (McIntosh et al. 2008; Valdez-Martinez et al. 2006); determining the social value of the research and dissemination of findings into policy change (Lairumbi et al. 2008); and securing the willing engagement of participants in research (Marsh et al. 2008). On the other hand, bioethics is thought to work as a lubricant enabling the rollout of neoliberal research practices. In other words, ethical oversight is present not so much to protect the participants as to facilitate certain kinds of research. Amit Prasad (2009) and Louise White (2011), for example, argue that consent, a keystone of bioethics, establishes a contract that works primarily in the interests of markets and the state and has little to do with autonomous decision making about research participation.

It is our aim to look beneath the normative conceptualizations of bioethics as discourse and to explore the considerable work being undertaken to make bioethics work in practice—that is, to make institutional forms fit, concepts intelligible, and values commensurable (see chapters 5 and 7). At this point, there might be the appearance of a smooth articulation of beliefs, values, and objectives, but closer examination reveals something rather more unruly and contingent. Interest in this encounter has led to a body of work that throws light on the tensions that occur when biomedical research is carried out in settings that are culturally and economically very different from those of Europe and North America. These tensions are not easily visible from the dominant perspectives of biomedicine and its accompanying ethics, which tend to assume the biomedical model they serve has spread in a uniform and consistent manner. This is an assumption that is beginning to come under closer scrutiny in the economically developing world (Chattopadhyay and De Vries 2013; Finkler 2000; Myser 2007, 2011). The emerging critique is one that demands the assumed underpinning "requirements" and "obligations" of experimental research be made explicit (Stengers 2010). Failure to do so is to risk perpetuating an epistemological exclusion and inferiorization.

Our own work seeks to extend these insights by connecting the assemblage of international biomedical research and its ethical governance to the values and practices of the society and culture in which it lands (see chapters 5 and 6). To this end, our analysis focuses on bioethics as immanent in the day-to-day practices of those who are involved in medical research—that is, as an *emic* rather than an *etic* category. To reiterate a distinction elaborated upon by Raymond De Vries, our interest is in an anthropology *of* bioethics, rather than an anthropology *for* or *in* bioethics (De Vries 2004; also see Hedgecoe 2004). We are interested in what it actually looks like from below, not what it is supposed to look like from above.

An anthropology of bioethics thus tries to show how the universal and normative protocols of biomedical research are rendered operative in local settings (Simpson 2004b). Critical in understanding this move is how diverse beliefs and values play out in everyday research practices, or as "ordinary ethics," to use Michael Lambek's term: "Human beings cannot avoid being subject to ethics, speaking and acting with ethical consequences, evaluating our actions and those of others, acknowledging and refusing acknowledgement, caring and taking care, but also being aware of the failure to do so consistently" (2010, 1). It is out of the "failure to do so consistently" that different registers of what might be deemed "unethical" practice open up and find expression: from the personal and interpersonal through to the organizational and macropolitical. For example, developing an appropriate "research culture" involves resources that have to be won in the face of competition and be managed and disbursed by groups and individuals operating according to social, cultural, and political realities as they exist on the ground. In these routine realities, the discourse of bioethics offers new ways of articulating and framing existing concerns about fairness, equity, discrimination, and a host of other ways in which the ordinariness of the unethical are addressed in practice.

Here our ethnography takes us farther into a world of conversation, argument, and dispute about how biomedical research might articulate the wider objectives of economic and health development as conceived locally (see chapter 8). These are profoundly ethical questions and moreover ones that often fall outside the accepted scope of bioethics. The ways in which the ordinariness of ethics (and the unethical) is woven into experimental practice thus becomes crucial for understanding how clinical trials operate as a conduit through which material, economic, and intellectual resources might find their way into local settings.

To develop our anthropology of bioethics, clinical trials, and international collaboration, we bring together ethnographic research performed in Sri Lanka across a range of biomedical research settings for over a decade. More specifically, we followed the work of two research organizations. One was based in a university and performed research in collaboration with a pharmaceutical company, and the other was a charitably funded research group performing research with more of a public health focus. We were thus able to follow trials of two different kinds. Our ethnographic account of these trials in chapters 2 and 3 provides the groundwork for the elaboration of conceptual and second order developments that are taken up in the anthropology of bioethics, which takes up the second half of the book.

Structure of the Book

The objective of this book is threefold. First, we describe ethnographically and historically international collaborations in biomedical research from a low-income setting. Second, we document the ways in which projects conceived at a global scale are accomplished practically and conceptually at the local level. And third, we explore the unintended as well as the intended consequences of these accomplishments.

In chapters 2, 3, and 4 we provide an account of clinical trials in Sri Lanka and the backdrop against which they are taking place. In chapter two, "Collaborating in Context," we give brief histories of biomedicine, biomedical research, and medical and bioethics in Sri Lanka. In the second part of the chapter, we also describe our entry into the field of biomedical research in Sri Lanka. We reflect upon our role as collaborators studying collaboration and the consequences this role has for the production of ethnographic description.

In chapters 3 and 4 we give detailed accounts of the two trials we observed during our research. These were both identified as important examples of research initiatives that were carried out in Sri Lanka, but they introduced significant elements from outside in terms of personnel, procedures, and the capacity to successfully perform the trial. They were thus seen as being in some sense "international." Moreover, although social studies of clinical trials have tended to follow the conduct of one particular trial (e.g. Brives 2016; Le Marcis 2015; Montgomery and Pool 2017), we are able to situate the trials we studied within a wider "landscape of collaboration" and within the historical development of biomedical research in Sri Lanka. The inclusion of this comparative and longer-term dimension enables us to reflect on how trials become configured in the quest to meet broader objectives and aspirations than the scientific questions answered in the particular trials.

In chapter 3 we present the Joint Pain Trial. This study was a randomized, placebo-controlled, double-blind, multicenter, phase 2 trial of a novel compound for the relief of joint pain. It was conducted at the Clinical Trials Unit of the Human Genetics Unit in the Medical Faculty of the University of Colombo, was funded by a foreign pharmaceutical company, and was monitored by an Indian contract research organization (CRO). The trial aimed at gaining FDA approval for a compound that would most likely find its way into Western rather than Sri Lankan markets. There were, however, plans for post-trial access for the trial's participants. Similar products were already in international markets but were not available in Sri Lanka.

In chapter 4 we present the Paraquat Poisoning Trial. This was also a randomized, placebo-controlled, double-blind, phase 2 trial. The tested compound was cyclophosphamide, which has significant toxicity but has been approved as having an acceptable risk-benefit ratio for certain serious conditions and is available in the marketplace. There was low-level evidence that it would reduce early death due to severe pulmonary injury caused by paraquat poisoning, and the trial in question was established to test this systematically. Unlike the Joint Pain Trial, this study was designed to address a pressing local public health concern: paraquat poisoning among farmers. The study was aimed at preventing death through poisoning and, in addition to the clinical end points, improving general patient management and achieving a better understanding of the condition. The study, performed as part of a larger collaboration on clinical toxicology in South Asia, was funded by an international health research charity. The international partners of this research organization were researchers from India, Bangladesh, Australia, and the United Kingdom and laboratories in the United Kingdom, Portugal, and Australia, where some laboratory tests were also conducted.

At the end of chapter 4, we draw comparisons between the two trials and highlight the differences in how the trials were set up, configured, and managed. We show how differently funded trials not only operate with different objectives but have different dynamics in terms of the knowledge they produce and the practices that they operate with.

In chapters 5, 6, and 7 we consider how engagement with clinical trials assemblages results in the work of localization. In these chapters, we show that this work is not simply about the installation of infrastructure and implementing procedures but is also about second order conceptual change regarding ethics, persons, and practices. These aspects of change are central to our attempts to understand the relationship between biomedical research *and* development—but, more importantly, research *as* development. In chapter 5, we consider the way that the idea of the "human subject" is conceived of within biomedical research and the friction that this brings when taken up by doctors and researchers who have come through their training in Sri Lanka. In chapter 6, we return to the Joint Pain Trial. By way of an account of the running of the trial, we show the creative work that goes into running a trial that must, perforce, look like one running anywhere else in the world but is in fact one that must be operable in the local setting. In chapter 7, we document episodes from the Paraquat Poisoning Trial and how the participants are moved within the logic of the trial from being an abject (one who has self-harmed, is socially stigmatized, and is barely alive), to an object (a body that is the object of measurement), to a subject (a person who is accorded certain rights and status as a participant in a trial conducted to international standards).

In the first seven chapters, we are mostly interested in the voices that tell of a broad alignment between the interests of biomedical research and those of national development, whether this be seen in terms of economic or as health indices. In chapter 8, we present something of an antithesis to this view. There we describe a series of conflicts in which critical voices are heard raising the specter that collaboration of the warm type might be a masquerade for the cooler and more exploitative one. These cases prove to be very important for understanding the ongoing conversations that occur around clinical trials, bioethics, and collaboration in Sri Lanka and in which we find important clues as to how biomedical research in low-income settings operates in practice and what is at stake for those who are conducting the trials.

In our conclusion (chapter 9) we consider the unintended and intended consequences arising from international research collaboration. A key observation is that the collaborative accomplishment of the clinical trial, whether successful or not, does far more than its stated objectives in that it engages local actors at multiple levels—social, economic, cultural, and political. In this engagement, the basic currencies of scientific collaboration—research, ethics, randomized control trials, and the very idea of collaboration itself—are contingent and negotiated in practice. It is in this flux of experimentation and biomedical advance that research works in novel ways to generate change.

Chapter 2

Collaboration in Context

[Collaboration is] . . . human behavior that facilitates the sharing of meaning
and completion of activities with respect to a mutually shared superordinate
goal and which takes place in a particular social, or work, setting.

(Iivonen and Sonnenwald 2000, 79)

Science, like any other activity involving social collaboration,
is subject to shifting fortunes.

(Merton [1942] 1973)

The research collaborations that we focus on in this book all took place
in Sri Lanka, an island republic of some 20 million people off the southern
tip of India. This location forms the backdrop for our study of how biomedical research can become tangled with economic, infrastructural, epistemological, and scientific development. To understand the specificities of this entanglement by means of ethnographic enquiry in the present day, it is
necessary to begin with some sense of how things came to be as they are. In
this chapter we move through a series of layers en route to our own engagement with the field of clinical trials, collaboration, and bioethics. We provide concise histories of biomedicine, biomedical research, and the parallel
development of medical ethics, research ethics, and subsequently bioethics
in Sri Lanka. This historical overview sets the scene for our account of the
clinical trials that we observed. In the second half of the chapter we describe
how we as researchers entered into this context as both ethnographers and
collaborators. In a context so infused with the idea of collaboration, we had
to collaborate as well. We explore the implications of this simple methodolog-

ical fact for ethnographic work in this context and more generally for researching expert systems and professional practice.

Biomedicine in Sri Lanka

The tradition of biomedicine is very firmly established in Sri Lanka. The Civil Medical Department of the British colonial administration was first established as a department separate from the one dealing with the occupying military forces in 1858. Although aimed specifically at the control of smallpox, the creation of a department to address the health needs of the local population, as distinct from the needs of the colonizers, marked an important step on the road to a national health service (Uragoda 1987, 81). Nonetheless, historians of colonial medicine have noted a circularity in how it developed. As Margaret Jones put it, "Western scientific medicine in its tropical form, along with Western sanitary methods, were imposed on populations whose health problems largely stemmed from the exploitative drives of the metropolitan power in the first place" (Jones 2000, 88; see also Arnold 2000; Hewa 2012 on hookworm eradication). Investment in medical research was thus necessary, in the first instance, to preserve a reasonably healthy workforce.

The Colombo Medical School opened in 1870 and is the second oldest in Asia after the Calcutta Medical College in India which opened in 1848. The school developed a distinguished tradition of providing biomedical education to the local population. Teaching followed British curricula, and the degrees were verified from the United Kingdom. Any postgraduate medical training had to be obtained in the United Kingdom. The colonial backdrop is important for our efforts to understand how contemporary international collaborations work in Sri Lanka and elsewhere. Indeed, it is evident that Britain, Europe, and the colonies have been enmeshed in a complex network of exchanges over a long period. Similar to what we postulate analytically about research, Hormoz Ebrahimnejad, writing on the encounter between traditional and modern medicine in Iran, has argued that rather than a one-way diffusion from the latter to the former, there was, in fact, an ongoing circularity. Ebrahimnejad goes on to claim that Western medicine itself became modernized in the colonies rather than being exported to them in an already "modern" form (Ebrahimnejad 2009). Then as now, there were flows in both directions. As Mark Harrison has suggested, it would be mistaken to think that the colonial countries were excluded from knowledge production; many doctors made their careers in the colonies, which provided sites for research, experimentation, and innovation (Harrison 2010; see also Johnson and Khalid 2012; Raj 2013). Knowledge transfer between Britain and the colonies was thus possible through the networks that connected colonial medical practitioners and administrators and their metropolitan counterparts. The transfer of resources also played its part. Soma Hewa (1995), for example, has documented the role of the American Rockefeller Foundation in developing public health campaigns such as the one aimed at hookworm eradication among tea estate laborers between 1915 and 1920, which became an important platform upon which local public health services were eventually built.

Throughout the nineteenth and early twentieth centuries and until independence in 1948, Sri Lanka, or Ceylon as it was previously known, was considered a model colony within the British Empire. Local elites were highly Westernized and politically moderate, and the medical sector in particular had seen generations of collaborative interaction with "foreigners." Even today, the medical profession preserves a strong sense of identity modeled on the structures that took root during the British colonial period.

The Anglicization of medicine was, and continues to be, reinforced by the use of English as the medium of medical (and other professional) education. Indeed, the language issue remains a source of tension, as the majority of the population receive primary and secondary education in their mother tongue (Sinhala or Tamil) but then have to take their medical degrees in English. Furthermore, an entrenched Anglophone biomedicine has had the effect of marginalizing the indigenous systems of medicine. As Kamalika Pieris has noted, in the nineteenth century the discussions regarding the development of a medical school identified one of its aims as being to "send out well-educated young men to open up the dispensaries of the Island and to diffuse a knowledge of European medicine among the poorer classes of the community and [thereby] in time supersede the ignorant *vedarala*" (Pieris 2001, 17). The *vedarala* were native physicians practicing a variety of indigenous medical techniques, including Ayurveda, and antipathy toward them was well established among practitioners of biomedicine. Despite the efforts to reclaim and elevate indigenous traditions (Wickramasinghe 2014, 104), this antipathy has continued to manifest itself among some present-day doctors and researchers. For much of its history, the Sri Lankan medical profession has not only been highly Westernized, English-speaking, and of high status but also cut off from the beliefs and values about health and illness held by the majority of the population.

In more recent times, an inexorable shift toward deregulation and an open-market economy has shaped health care access. After the election in 1977 of J. R. Jayawardena, who led the government with an agenda of fundamental market reform and economic liberalization, the private sector has come to play an increasingly important role in health care. In 1978, for example, doctors were for the first time allowed to maintain private practices in addition to their government responsibilities, a development that spurred a spectacular growth in private provision, particularly in tertiary care. International, market-priced pharmaceuticals also became available (to those who could afford to pay for them). In an overview of the health care system, Dulitha N. Fernando argued that it is difficult to assess the exact contribution made by private health care providers as the sector is not regulated, but she estimated that approximately 50 percent of primary medical care in 2000 was provided by private sector general practitioners (Fernando 2001). The government sector has been further affected, particularly in primary care provision, as pressures from the World Bank and other international financial institutions have increasingly undermined the earlier patterns of welfare expenditure (Jayasinghe 2002, 6–7).[1] Furthermore, the import of equipment to private medical institutions was greatly accelerated after 1977 by the granting of duty-free concessions. The result of these and other developments has been an overall trend toward private medicine.

In contrast, the public sector, which to date has provided free health care at the point of need, has fallen further behind the private sector in some fields.[2] Steven Russell's investigation of health care in Sri Lanka provided further evidence for the widespread use of private medicine in Sri Lanka (2005). His study examined a wide range of income groups and concluded that government services, which continue to be provided free at the point of need, remain important. Despite the growth of private medicine, people do not choose their providers based on whether they have to pay for them or not. The interweaving of public and private sectors is now dense both in terms of users and providers. The turn to private medicine raises concerns that private provision might even displace the state as the key provider of health services altogether. The ability to respond to health care problems has been impeded by disjointed management of health matters, administration, and budgeting. For example, in writing about the impact of technology on health care, Abeykoon highlighted the "confusion and conflicts over roles, responsibilities and lines of accountability between central and provincial levels of the Ministry of Health" as a "major issue" that resulted from devolution after 1977 (Abeykoon 2003, 11). Saroj Jayasinghe and Nalaka Mendis also reported that the health care system was "fragmented" with poor processes and structure and "lacks data and reliable information" (2002, 100; also see Rannan-Eliya and Sikurajapathy 2009, 329–36). It is in an environment where health care costs rise inexorably and privatization seems to present itself at every turn that international medical collaborations are currently being assembled.

Yet, Sri Lanka is cited by many as a success story for having managed, despite low spending and gross domestic product, to run a free national health system (Bhutta, Nundy, and Abbasi 2004). Part of this health system was the Sri Lankan pharmaceutical policy regime set in place in the early 1970s (Cooray 2016). At the time, it was internationally groundbreaking. As one of these internationally trained scholars, the pharmacologist Senaka Bibile, who had studied in Sri Lanka and obtained his doctorate from the University of Edinburgh, devised a so-called Essential Medicines List for Sri Lanka. At the time, Sri Lanka depended on imports from the United States and Europe and suffered from prices that were too high for people to pay. The Bibile system consisted of a list of drugs that were considered crucial to the health of the population; these drugs were either bought in bulk by the local State Pharmaceutical Corporation or were manufactured locally and provided for free to patients in public hospitals. The list initially included only fifty-two pharmaceuticals, so drug availability was rather narrow, but these generics kept prices down (Lall 1977, 692). For example, with the institutionalizing of a state-regulated pharmaceutical sector, the prices for antibiotics dropped by 85 percent in 1972 even while they were rising elsewhere globally (Lall 1977). The World Health Organization (WHO) adopted the system, and a worldwide Essential Medicines List has been released every two years.

Successes in such areas as family planning, nutrition, and female literacy have helped bring about substantial increases in life expectancy. Rasika Jayasekara and Tim Schultz (2007) noted that Sri Lankan life expectancy increased from around forty-three years of age just before independence to seventy-three years in 2004. However, as people began to live longer, they in turn contributed to the increase of noncommunicable and degenerative diseases such as heart disease and diabetes (Ghaffar, Reddy, and Singhi 2004). Palitha Abeykoon (1998) estimated that in the twenty-five years between 1995 and 2020, the number of those aged sixty and older will have more than doubled in Sri Lanka. As such, the problems that affect the elderly—such as falls, depression, cognitive dysfunction, and severe visual impairment—are set to increase significantly (Weerasuriya and Jayasinghe 2005, cited in Jayasekara and Schultz 2007). Jayasekara and Schultz also suggested that social and demographic changes have resulted in a weakening of "traditional and extended family networks"; younger generations becoming more dispersed and parental generations becoming more isolated has put further pressure on the health care system (Jayasekara and Schultz 2007; Widger and Kabir, n.d.). Moreover, noncommunicable diseases are on the rise at a time when the country is still managing infectious diseases as well as those rooted in poverty such as maternal anemia, stunted growth, and childhood malnutrition (Abeykoon 2003). As such, the health care system is forced to "fight on two different fronts" (Gunawardene 1999), and these conditions weigh heavily on the resources available in Sri Lanka (Deshapriya and Welikala 2004; Jayasekara and Schultz 2007). As we will see in chapter 3, this emerging epidemiological profile is important for international research collaborations: the increasing convergence with populations in the West opens the possibility for new populations of human subjects to participate in externally sponsored trials, and it is into this setting that the research collaborations we describe in this book were introduced.

Finally, it is impossible to give an overview of contemporary health care provision in Sri Lanka without reference to the communal and political violence that has consumed the island in recent decades. Over twenty-five years of conflict between the Liberation Tigers of Tamil Eelam (LTTE) and the government of Sri Lanka has taken a major toll on health and public services (Siriwardhana and Wickramage 2014). The bulk of fieldwork for this study was conducted during the time leading up to the end of the war, a very tense, oppressive era. Ongoing stressful living conditions and fear of deadly attacks and more silent dangers such as landmines were the norm for much of the population (Reilley, Abeyasinghe, and Pakianathar 2002). The war and internal population displacement placed great strain on hospital beds and services with the increased number of people suffering from long-term mental and physical health problems and physical disabilities. These conditions have left Sri Lanka facing significant challenges for both delivering health care and conducting research. When it comes to improving health care and developing infrastructure, powerful humanitarian and economic imperatives are at work, to which international research collaborations might speak. In documenting the practices of such collaborations, we describe the novel strategies at work to effect transformative change on the wider health system in Sri Lanka. This points to not only material changes but also conceptual ones, in which research, evidence, and experimentation begin to figure as essential drivers of policy formulation and change. In the next section, we provide a brief overview of past biomedical research in Sri Lanka as a necessary prelude to our discussion of contemporary research collaborations.

Biomedical Research in Sri Lanka

When international collaborations are conducted in Sri Lanka, they do not occur in an empty epistemic space. As we have seen, layers of interaction and exchange already existed that had built up over many centuries. Within this complex mosaic, local scholars will also proudly draw attention to Sri Lanka's own traditions of medical research. Medieval ayurvedic physicians are credited with having developed early surgical techniques; their attempts at rhinoplasty to repair facial disfigurement and techniques for repairing anal fistula have been documented (Aluwihare 1982). More recent times also have seen medical advances, particularly in the fields of surgery and management of tropical diseases. For example, Pieris referred to the mid-nineteenth-century surgeon P. D. Antonisz being lauded for performing the first successful esophagotomy and ovariotomy (Pieris 2001, 129). Trials carried out by local doctors have included a trial to test a cure for hookworm, in which patients were randomly selected from local hospitals (Goodwin, Jayewardene, and Standen 1958). Pieris also referred to a report in the *Journal of the Ceylon Branch of the British Medical Association* describing a trial performed at the general hospital using morphine and hyoscine as anesthetics during labor (Pieris 2001, 132). Other notable interventions in the field of experimental trials included one of the first trials of the contraceptive pill in the 1950s, which led Darshi Thoradeniya to describe Sri Lanka as a "laboratory for pill trials" (forthcoming).

Despite this history of experimentation, scientific research using randomized controlled trials in Sri Lanka has been limited. In a global survey of science capacity calculated according to networks of collaboration, international and national publications, and availability of funds for research, Sri Lanka landed fifth from bottom in a list of seventy-five countries (Wagner 2008, 132). This result led Caroline Wagner to describe Sri Lanka as one of a number of countries that was scientifically "lagging" (Wagner 2008). Although, as Amit Prasad (2014) reminds, it is important to treat such surveys with caution, they also serve a particular rhetorical purpose in justifying capacity-building activities.

In numerous essays and talks published over the last two decades, the eminent Sri Lankan microbiologist Professor S. N. Arseculeratne has maintained a scathing critique of the state of scientific research in his native Sri Lanka and provided his own views of why more developments have not been made (Arseculeratne 1999, 2008). In Arseculeratne's view, the problem stems not from any global economic or political disparities but from a widespread deficiency in the way that science is promoted and understood in Sri Lanka. He describes a kind of scientific malaise that runs through the major teaching and research institutes. He sees this as particularly evident in the way that medical education is delivered. Medical doctors are not expected to publish research to progress in their careers; for university researchers, publication expectations are low or nonexistent. One of Arseculeratne's main criticisms is that medical education is largely based on factual recall and rarely encourages analytical, experimental, or creative approaches. In one of his talks, he spoke of medicine needing to be seen "not merely as a craft with utilitarian ends, but as an important component of science with an intellectual background that includes the history and philosophy of modern science" (Arseculeratne 2010).

According to Arseculeratne, an unfortunate corollary of this deeply engrained utilitarianism is that the curiosity that drives medical research and innovation is only weakly present in Sri Lanka. He sees a further inhibitor of young doctors' curiosity in the authoritarian ethos of medical education and practice. For medical students, relationships are marked by strong vertical hierarchies based on the status, knowledge, charisma, and reputation of their teachers. The steep power gradients that separate junior medical staff from their superiors manifest in a good deal of fear, a concern to avoid offence, and a tendency to replicate rather than challenge received wisdom; to fall foul of a powerful senior is to risk long-lasting damage to one's reputation and future prospects. Such conditions are hardly conducive to a free and open exchange of ideas that challenges orthodoxy and generates innovative approaches.

Given the problems faced by the health sector in Sri Lanka, it is hardly surprising that researcher malaise has been further compounded by starved research budgets and a significant drain of expertise out of the country. These factors go some considerable way to explaining why Sri Lanka has been pronounced scientifically lagging.

In contrast to the view of the rote-learning medics practicing in an enfeebled research environment, Sri Lankan medical students are also pointed toward a venerable tradition in which local doctors working in resource-poor settings overcome tremendous odds by using their ingenuity and skills of improvisation. As Pieris put it in her history of the Sri Lankan medical profession, "the dedicated government doctor could be described as possessed of a perpetual pioneering spirit in that the government service invariably held shortcomings which the doctors had to somehow overcome if they were to deliver a satisfactory service" (Pieris 2001, 139). In contemporary settings, doctors still have to be able to perform with limited diagnostic testing facilities and make decisions drawing on basic clinical expertise, judgment, and experience. The heroic image of the doctor that medical students are taught to emulate is that of the healer, who brings relief from suffering in the service of others and without thought of material gain—a benevolent, paternalistic role that has particularly powerful resonances within Sri Lankan culture beyond medicine.[3]

The reason for this brief excursion into Sri Lankan biomedical traditions is that it provides some sense of what was there before and what some would see as an impediment to change. As we will discuss in chapter 6, the extant research culture and efforts to transform it through international collaboration result in a reshaping of the subjectivities that underpin many of the roles and relationships that feature in the practice of biomedicine. In particular we focus on the relationship between doctor and patient, and the ways in which new modes of acting and being are informed by the relationship between researcher and research participant. This transformation, however, is only partially wrought through practice. Another significant source of such transformation is found in the systems of research governance that the new modes of experimental research bring with them. In the next section we provide, by way of backdrop, a brief history of the rise of research ethics and regulation in Sri Lanka.

Research Governance in Sri Lanka

In developing world settings, biomedicine and biomedical research not only have become increasingly imbricated with each other but are both now shaped by the demands of research governance and regulation. This is particularly the case where human participants are involved. The shift from a physician-cum-scientist virtue-based ethics to one in which there is externalized evidence of ethical intent captured through audit and contract is in many respects readable from the rise of ethics reviews by committee. In the most basic of terms, the approval of a formally constituted body of experts in the form of an ethics review committee (ERC) is intended to ensure that research is beneficial, scientifically valid, and above all safe for those who participate (Stark 2011). At the time that our research was carried out, the machinery for ethics review was being rapidly developed across South Asia, with ERCs following a broadly similar institutional and procedural format to those established in Europe and the United States (Douglas-Jones 2012).

The genealogy underpinning these developments is well established. The principles of ethics review, as laid out in the Declaration of Helsinki (World Medical Association 2013, paragraph 23), include the need for a clearly formulated research protocol as well as information about funding, sponsors, institutional affiliations, conflicts of interest, and the use of incentives for participants. When the research is to take place in a country different from that of the research sponsor, it is expected that there will be a local ethics review based on the Helsinki principles, or what is generally referred to as a "two-ended review." The European Medicines Agency (EMA) has emphasized the need for local ethics committees even more strongly, insisting that a local ethics committee is a prerequisite for a clinical trial to take place at all (European Medicines Agency 2012; CIOMS 2016, 29–31). The Universal Declaration on Bioethics and Human Rights takes these requirements one stage further, toward research as (a catalyst for) development—the focus of our interest here. Article 19, which deals with the topic of ERCs, states the following:

> Independent, multidisciplinary and pluralist ethics committees should be established, promoted and supported at the appropriate level in order to a) assess the relevant ethical, legal and scientific and social issues related to research projects involving human beings, b) provide advice on ethical

problems in clinical settings, c) assess scientific and technological developments, formulate recommendations and contribute to the preparation of
guidelines on issues within the scope of this Declaration and d) foster debate,
education and public awareness of, and engagement in, bioethics. (UNESCO
2005, Article 19)

Here the remit extends beyond the mere setting of standards and begins to
move into the realms of capacity building and the creation of a climate in
which the objectives of the Universal Declaration will be realized. The encouragement for economically developed countries to grow local capacity in
research governance is typically expressed in terms of empowerment and the
hope that various forms of ethical imperialism can be mitigated. The involvement of host-country ethics committees in research governance also brings
into play their knowledge and experience of local conditions, which it is believed will facilitate the research and benefit its participants.

However, a number of problems are usually identified in the development
of the two-ended ethics review model. As Ruth Macklin pointed out, the tie-
up between the ends often leaves much to be desired; even though it is now
common to have host and sponsor engaged in ethics review, there are few
link-ups between ERCs and little by way of significant and potentially productive exchange (Macklin 2004, 152). Concerns have been expressed about
the competence of local bodies to review research in a way that is broadly
equivalent to the sponsor country's procedures. Questions also arise when host
and sponsor country ethics committees appear to work with fundamentally
different ethical standards and principles. Such discrepancies have been the
case in a number of clinical trials where local committees, after full ethics
review of a project, appeared to be prepared to accept standards much lower
than would pass in economically developed countries. Paul Farmer goes further still, identifying these discrepancies as the tacit acceptance within
international biomedical research of fundamental health inequalities between low- and high-income countries (Farmer 2004, 200; see also Geissler
2013). He suggested that structural differences are at times read as "cultural" differences and dismissed as acceptable local practices.

Notwithstanding these concerns, ERCs are now a ubiquitous feature of
research governance. During the period covered by our research, many Sri
Lankan doctors and academics were fervently engaged in capacity building in bioethics, specifically in relation to research ethics and governance

(Douglas-Jones 2012). The reasons were simple: without corresponding local review procedures, the experimental research activity taking place in Sri Lanka would not be recognized as part of the global episteme of ethically validated knowledge production. In other words, the opportunities for international collaboration would be severely limited, and with this would come the kind of epistemic exclusion discussed in the introduction.

Partly in response to the potential loss of opportunity, between 1980 and 2006 the number of ERCs in Sri Lanka rose steadily from two to fifteen. At the time of our research in 2010, the figure was twenty, with more planned. Ethics committees were established in the universities of Colombo (1981), Peradeniya (early 1980s), Galle (1984), Jaffna (1985), and Kelaniya (1995) as well as the Sri Lanka Medical Association national committee (1999) (Dissanayake, Mendis, and Lanerolle 2006). According to local commentators, in the 1990s training in medical ethics was badly in need of updating and development in response to scientific and technological advances in biomedical sciences and to the changing structure of health care delivery. Vajira Dissanayake, N. Mendis, and R. D. Lanerolle (2006) described the transition as being from a well-established medical ethics concerned essentially with the conduct of doctors in relation to their patients to one that was more closely aligned with the directives of a global bioethics.

In 2007, the Forum of Ethics Committees Sri Lanka drafted a guideline: "Ethics Review Committee Guidelines: A Guide for Developing Standard Operating Procedures for Committees That Review Biomedical Proposals." This document was intended to unify the island's diverse procedures in the context of ethics reviews. The direction of travel was at that time strongly influenced by a widely read article by Ezekiel Emanuel, David Wendler, and Christine Grady (2000) entitled "What Makes Clinical Research Ethical?" This article has been influential in providing ethics committees in the developing world with a checklist of sorts when it comes to dealing with outside collaborations. Although this national guideline now exists for Sri Lanka, many committees have in fact developed their own standard operating procedures, rendering the landscape of ethics review quite diverse.

Capacity-building initiatives around ethics review and research governance in Sri Lanka have drawn strong support from medical elites keen to engage with the opportunities that international research collaboration makes possible (see Douglas-Jones 2012). This support has resulted in the opening up of new institutional spaces in which novel forms of advocacy and activism are evident. Support for local capacity-building initiatives has come from organizations such as the Forum for Ethical Review Committees in Asia and the Western Pacific (FERCAP), the Strategic Initiative for Developing Capacity in Ethical Review (SIDCER), and the Global Forum on Bioethics (GFB), all of which signal the bioethical collaborations which necessarily underpin scientific collaboration. Affiliation to these organizations and the establishment of local branches (for example, FERC–Sri Lanka) has been an important route to harmonization and the dissemination of good practice. It is also a way for local researchers to connect with regional networks and to participate in transnational research assemblages. For example, the Colombo Medical Faculty committee has had access to training from the U.S. National Institutes of Health located in Bethesda, Maryland. A researcher from the faculty has completed a bioethics degree there, and bioethics lectures have been streamed to students. The Colombo Medical Faculty Ethics Committee is also accredited by the Strategic Initiative for Developing Capacity in Ethical Review (SIDCER), an initiative which emerged out of collaboration between the WHO and the Special Programme for Research and Training in Tropical Diseases (TDR). At the time of writing, no other ethics committee in Sri Lanka had this accreditation. The National Science Foundation, whose ethics committee authorizes applications that have national reach, has developed its provision through training provided by UNESCO. Finally, only eight out of the twenty ethics committees operating in the country at the time of this writing are accredited by the Sri Lankan Drug Regulatory Authority to give ethics clearance to clinical trials. These ERCs were in the University of Colombo, University of Kelaniya, University of Sri Jayewardenapura, University of Peradeniya, University of Ruhuna, University of Jaffna, the Sri Lanka Medical Association, and the Medical Research Institute. As we will see in chapter 8, awareness of the regulatory landscape is important when it comes to understanding the internal debates and positions that are thrown up when bioethics and research governance are addressed in the local context.

Arguably, however, when it comes to clinical trials regulations, most ERCs follow the latest version of the International Conference on Harmonization Good Clinical Practice Guidelines (ICH-GCP). These guidelines provide an authoritative summary of good practice for industry-funded clinical trials from the European Union, Japan, the United States, and, more recently, from Australia, Canada, the Nordic countries, and WHO. These widely used guidelines aim to provide "a more economical use of human, animal and material resources, and the elimination of unnecessary delay in the global development and availability of new medicines whilst maintaining safeguards on quality, safety and efficacy, and regulatory obligations to protect public health" (Dixon 1998). ERCs are thus required to abide by an evolving corpus of principles and practice guidelines and render these operative in local settings. The need to be trained in all these aspects of research governance is a source of considerable capacity-building endeavor. Rachel Douglas-Jones (2012), in a study of capacity building for ERCs across Asia, has drawn attention to the significance of standard operating procedures (SOPs). She showed how, by using a locally adopted template of SOPs, ERCs are able to avoid the challenge of managing cultural specificity in the face of universal values.

In addition to universities and hospitals, promotion of bioethics has also taken place in the nongovernmental sector. The Institute for Research and Development (IRD) is a nongovernmental organization of local doctors who, drawing on their own networks of international facilitators, run their own training workshops. The IRD is primarily geared to promoting the link between scientific research and development but doing so in a way that fully recognizes the power differentials that plague this relationship. Bioethics is one of the discourses adopted to analyze and critique this relationship. Members of this group produced their own take on developing world bioethics in the book *Research Ethics from a Developing World Perspective* (Sumathipala and Siribaddana 2003). This was the first attempt in Sri Lanka to complement, with local voices, the vast corpus of Western-facing commentaries on the ethics of biomedical research. The book draws attention to the absence of ethics guidelines for research in Sri Lanka as well as the need to engage with the fundamental inequalities that characterize health research in the global south.

At one end of the spectrum of local concerns for the need for bioethics lie prosaic concerns about the protection of vulnerable subjects and the belief that the discipline of bioethics can provide some leverage on this issue. For example, the recruitment of local participants to international clinical trials has produced a range of justifications, rationales, excuses, explanations, and accusations of exploitation and has on occasion resulted in trials being closed down because of concerns about their actual or potential harm to the participants. The IRD has been vociferous in raising such concerns and has drawn on bioethics discourses as a way of highlighting exploitation while at the same time promoting local scientific research as integral to development in Sri Lanka.[4]

At the other end of the spectrum, however, is a rhetoric of bioethics that addresses the novel technologies that are arriving in Sri Lanka. In addition to international clinical trials, these technologies include transplant surgery, gene technology, and assisted reproductive technologies, all of which raise questions about the limits of medical intervention as well as issues of access and equality.[5] These biomedical and technological advancements create another conduit for particular kinds of bioethics discourses to enter into Sri Lanka. Local doctors and scientists want to show that they are progressive not only in science but also in the ethics by which the science is evaluated and governed. Having ethics expertise in place plays an important role in demonstrating to international audiences that Sri Lanka is on a par with most recent developments elsewhere. Here, ethics has the role of both facilitating possible future research and operating as a mode of protection. Where external audiences are concerned, there is anxiety that charges of ethical laxity or deficiency might be indexed to estimations of national development and scientific credibility.

All these activities, although local in their implementation, are underpinned by international funding. They also involve a great deal of movement of personnel into and out of the country for training and dissemination events, and they result in publications in international medical journals (e.g. Dissanayake, Mendis, and Lanerolle 2006; Sumathipala et al. 2003; Sumathipala, Siribaddana, and Patel 2004). In short, capacity building in bioethics is not simply a context that is created to receive new kinds of knowledge and expertise; it is thoroughly enmeshed in international exchanges (Simpson et al. 2015). The complexities that underlie the apparently simple objective of "capacity building" are further evident in the emergence of diverging lines of argument among different interlocutors in the discourses around bioethics in Sri Lanka.

Next we turn to an account of how we positioned ourselves—or rather were positioned—within biomedical research and international collaboration as a field of anthropological enquiry. We were dealing with people who had clear ideas and insights about the worlds in which they lived and which we attempted to participate in. Entanglement in this agenda meant that there were various points at which our research practices folded back on the contexts we were attempting to study. We were engaged in mutual knowledge making regarding bioethics and clinical trials, and spaces opened up for dialogue and collaborative reflection. The points where different collaborative intentions meet are not just about access—they have fundamental epistemological and ontological implications for the way that ethnography is formulated and produces its effects.

Converging Traditions of Collaboration

Collaboration has become a key paradigm when it comes to thinking about how scientific research should be conceptualized and organized.[6] The rhetoric of collaboration would suggest that working together across disciplines and research groupings produces important synergies: improving access to, and use of, equipment and resources (Wray 2002); bringing together complementary scientific competences resulting in shared access to samples, data, and equipment (Melin 2000, 34); providing novel solutions to problems (Thagard 2006); arriving at more reliable results (Fallis 2006); and achieving greater efficiencies in research practice and knowledge transfer (Beaver and Rosen 1978, 1979a, 1979b). As we will see later in this chapter, this paradigm has also opened up spaces for social scientists to engage in collaboration with scientists.

In the foregoing account of Sri Lankan biomedicine, research and governance and relations with foreign researchers and agencies are widely evident. Now we turn to another question: What does it mean to situate ourselves ethnographically within this ongoing flow of collaborative engagement? Carrying out ethnographic research among those undertaking international collaborative research activities initiated reflection on our own position as researchers and the epistemologies we were drawing upon. Working with this particular community of highly educated and critically reflexive informants inevitably shaped the character of the research we undertook. We could not take a "view from nowhere," and we ourselves became collaborators of a kind, with collaboration becoming central to our methodological engagement with the field.

As with the notion of para-ethnography, developed by George E. Marcus and Douglas Holmes, we were concerned to find more appropriate ways of acknowledging the character of fieldwork in settings in which science and a technocratic ethos are central (Holmes and Marcus 2008a; see also Marcus 2013). As Holmes and Marcus put it, "these [para-ethnographic] experiments speak to a particular problem: How do we pursue our inquiry when our subjects are themselves engaged in intellectual labors that resemble approximately or are entirely indistinguishable from our own methodological practice?" (Holmes and Marcus 2008b, 595–97). The description of para-ethnographic moments at various points in this analysis identifies the subjects of our enquiry as people who reflect and creatively theorize about their own work and worlds—thus, we are dealing with "counterparts" rather than "others" (Marcus 2013). The relationship we aspire to is thus not one in which there is a crude extraction of data but one in which we ourselves are engaged in collaborative relationships and epistemic partnerships. As Monica Konrad (2012) suggests, however, to study collaboration is to open up novel questions of positionality within the ethnographic endeavor—what are we to make of "collaborators collaborating"? Working *in* collaboration *on* collaboration is a radical departure for classical single-authored anthropological fieldwork. What consequences do "epistemic communities" composed of highly trained scientists and researchers hold for the conduct of ethnographic research (Heckler and Russell 2008)?

One important response to this question is that studying others going about the business of collaboration necessarily requires us to be drawn into particular kinds of relationships with them. Carried in on the back of the anthropologists' own version of collaboration—a willingness to engage constructively with the local scene—we encountered another kind of collaborative intent coming the other way, as we ourselves became conscripted as collaborators. Before actually beginning our part of the International Science and Bioethics Collaboration (ISBC) project research in Sri Lanka, it was necessary to make formal approaches to the institutions and groups with which we hoped to work. Having secured ethics approval from the review boards of Cambridge and Durham universities, with which the project was affiliated, it was necessary to obtain local approval in Sri Lanka.

For many of the Sri Lankan medical researchers with whom we went on to work, the idea of a review board in the United Kingdom giving approval for research that would go on in another country seemed inherently problematic. Thus, it came as no surprise that we were asked to submit an application for ethics review to a local ethics committee. Applying for this approval signaled particular collaborative intent and shaped how our intentions were to be grafted onto local networks. At the time, the clearance had to come from a medical ERC because our study was seen to be focusing on matters of health, even if by proxy. Moreover, at that time the local social science departments did not have any ethics committees. However, working without ethics clearance was not viewed as an option for us by our medical collaborators, who were building up expectations that having ethics clearance was mandatory for outsiders wanting to carry out research in Sri Lanka.

The form we completed was lengthy. Most of the items on it were geared to biomedical research and the collection of samples, so "n/a" (not applicable) was our most frequent response. It also required us to specify what, how, where, who, and how many we were going to study, in ways that implied levels of natural science, experimental prescience, and control that do not sit well with an ethnographic approach (Simpson 2011). Nonetheless, the form was important evidence that detailed who and what we were about, yet one element of the transaction made us think further about our local relations. Section 3.3.2.1 of the Ethics Committee Guidelines for Sri Lanka specifies that 1) a local collaborator (coinvestigator) from Sri Lanka with equal responsibility is essential, and 2) a written agreement regarding the sample/data ownership publication strategy (including issues such as authorship and the right of the Sri Lankan collaborator to publish data pertaining to Sri Lanka) and intellectual property rights should be in place (FERCSL 2007). It was clear that without the ERC's approval our research could not progress—a local imprimatur was essential.

Even though we upheld the collaborative prospect and saw value in a shared process, some of these notions did not fit with our ideas about ethnography as a way of working with others to understand their social and cultural practices. On the one hand, we were not "recruiting" people for a study in the strict sense of the term, nor did we see our questions as "interventions" being rolled out. Nor did we know exactly in advance who we were going to work with or how we were going to proceed. We also were concerned that collaboration might compromise our academic freedom in some way. In short, as social anthropologists, we found these ethics forms moving us into a rather unfamiliar methodological territory.

We discussed our concerns with our main contact-cum-gatekeeper-cum-collaborator, and we were reassured that the form was really to protect against "other kinds of researchers"—namely, those who come from the global north to prospect and extract without due reward or recognition for local researchers, who at worst act in ways that harm local populations. The specter of the unethical researcher loomed large in local discourses, particularly where foreign researchers were concerned. The history of serious exploitation by outsiders has been too long and too flagrant for this not to be the case. Although it was made clear to us that we were not seen as falling into this category, we nonetheless had to fill in the forms. No doubt it was a precautionary measure, just in case we turned out to be something other than what we appeared—in case we turned out to be just the same as all those others. The form did indeed cause much anxiety, particularly for Rachel Douglas-Jones who, as a doctoral student engaging in first-time fieldwork, was in a rather different relationship with her collaborators.

Ultimately, once they were completed and successfully reviewed, the forms were never referred to again. In many respects, the documents and the process of review functioned more as a public legitimation of our relationship with our collaborators than as an evaluation of the potential of our research to cause harm to our subjects. In short, the ethics review for this particular research was as much about marking the relationships that the research would initiate as it was about the protection of those who would participate in it. From the outset, collaboration was folded into our research in ways that would shape and prescribe both what we researched and how we could go about it. This was not fieldwork as we had known it (Clifford and Marcus 1986; Faubion and Marcus 2009; Marcus 2005; Rabinow et al. 2008; Westbrook 2009).

The vectors of our own collaborative tradition did not entirely meet with those of the people we wished to carry out research among. As Holmes and Marcus put it, "the ethnographer is a figure whose presence is anticipated" (2008a, 86); that is, there was a further dimension to our inculcation as collaborators. In this process of ethics clearance, we ourselves were subject to a counter-subjectification with its own ethics justification, not least of which was to make our interests visible. Taking this proposition seriously involved a shift in attention from our reflexive concerns to the uses of collaboration as an idiom to place us in somebody else's world. This is hardly surprising given that Sri Lankan society is one in which hierarchy, status, competition, and professional jealousy have to be negotiated on a daily basis. The idea of an objective and unattached researcher moving between different factions and interest groups was not only unrealistic but unfeasible. Incorporation into one part of the network necessarily precluded closeness to another part of it—

you have to choose your camp and, in so doing, understand what it is that is obscured as well as what this makes visible (Simpson 2006). In other words, that we had to collaborate should be seen alongside a rather more important observation: we were granted access in order to be collaborators, and collaboration was inevitable to conduct this research.

This way of looking at ethnographic fieldwork makes visible a particular set of dynamics concerning power and exchange. In a resource-constrained setting, collaboration with overseas researchers was seen to bring a number of benefits, both material and symbolic. It is, in effect, an attempt to reverse the process of draining away intellectual and human capital that continually undermines local efforts to create sustainable scientific communities. The passivity and distance that belies the designation "informant" thus gives way to creative attempts by local scientists and doctors to realize collaboration as something tangible and beneficial rather than merely rhetorical. From the perspective of our "subjects," the question that might be asked is, What, if anything, is to be gained as we enter into the assemblage of international social science research?

Some of the answers to this question clearly point to instrumental strategies. We have been asked by our collaborators at various points to provide input in ways that blur the boundary between research and practice and on occasion took us beyond our expertise and capability (such as the request for us to advise and help run a master's course in bioethics, supervise MPhil students, and help with PhD applications). Other requests, however, lay more in the realm of dialogue and the exchange of ideas about objects of common interest and concern. This included inputs into the supervision of local students who might not otherwise have access to social science perspectives on biomedicine, the coauthoring of publications, and the presentation of talks and seminars for local consumption.

Our subsequent attempts to think through the complex mesh of relationships in which we found ourselves operating was helped considerably by what transpired at a meeting held in the United Kingdom at which a group of social scientists came together to share their experiences of working with biomedical scientists.[7] The workshop, called "How Do We Collaborate?," and the discussions held in that meeting were reported in the journal *Biosocieties* (Prainsack et al. 2010). The nub of the issue was that in Europe, the United Kingdom, and the United States there is a growing tendency to include social scientists in projects that were hitherto strongly, and often exclusively, marked as the preserve of biomedical scientists. The rise of the "ethical, legal and social implications (ELSI) of science" agenda,[8] for example, has provided a widely accepted formulation of why purely scientific forms of expertise and practice need to be complemented by other kinds. The "How Do We Collaborate?" meeting was productive in enabling social science researchers from a range of disciplines to share insights and air frustrations and difficulties when working with professionals who are 1) practicing scientists and therefore themselves researchers, 2) interested in the representations that might be created about them and their practices, and 3) potentially in a position to exercise varying degrees of influence or "objection" (cf. E. Simpson 2016)—as stakeholders, users, and collaborators—over the conduct and outcomes of a research project. The workshop opened up many important issues arising from the engagement between social and biomedical scientists: identifying confusion, peer relations, objectivity, space for criticality, and the problem of "going native," to name but a few. Many of these issues seemed to be made visible because of a particular kind of framing. This effect was apparent in the eventual write-up, in which the day's discussions were parceled into sections: "getting access," "inside the field," and "outside the field" (Prainsack et al. 2010).

The day's initial discussions addressed the premise that social scientists collaborate with life scientists and medical researchers to get access to their studies, but once access has been granted the social scientists may be faced with compromising situations and trade-offs to retain their inside position and "positive relations with informants" (Prainsack et al. 2010, 281). In reflecting on how to manage these relations, especially after fieldwork has ended and when interpretations in publications may be questioned or vetoed, the discussion suggested that predetermined contracts or codes for mutual rights and duties, even when difficult due to the emergent and creative line of work, may mitigate problems in expectations.

This way of framing the research encounter is only helpful up to a point, and it barely addresses the complexities we are keen to explicate here. The main concern is that this conceptualization smuggles in traces of an objectivity that reifies the role and identity of the social science researcher within the collaboration. Framing the discussion in terms of "getting access" and being "inside or outside" casts the researcher as a kind of double agent who can enter, collect data, and exit with a snatched fragment of reality. The language of "informants" and "collaboration" seems troublingly consistent with the cooler themes of collaborative engagement (as we discussed in chapter 1).

In the crisis of representation that has unfolded in anthropology since the 1970s, there has been what Marcus Schlecker and Eric Hirsch describe as "an increasing erosion of the idea that any perspective could adequately capture an 'out-there reality'" (2001, 77). When attempting to study communities of experts and professionals, the intertwining of knowledge production between "those who are being studied" and "those who study" brings into question the assumption of *us* and *them* that is implicit in this way of framing the field. The problem is further compounded when the biomedical practices and domains we are seeking to study are located outside the global north. When operating beyond the well-documented and well-represented institutions of the America and Europe, the conceptual tools of *culture* and *society* that are used to study such encounters seem badly worn and run into considerable difficulties (Anderson 2009).

In reflecting on our own collaborative engagement with the world of biomedical research in Sri Lanka, we are perhaps beginning to move toward arrangements in which the social science researcher is rendered analytically visible and his or her role is not limited simply to working out the ethical, legal, and social implications (ELSI) of scientific research (see also Balmer et al. 2015). The rhetorical engagement of *science* and *society* into which social scientists are now being drawn (here, read "needing to do/have impact, to disseminate to stakeholders and end-users, to engage with publics of science, and, indeed, to collaborate") opens new possibilities and constraints when it comes to ethnographies of scientific research.

A further layer to this analysis was our collaboration as anthropologists. The "self" doing the analysis was not a customary single author—we were, in fact, already a crowd. It is to this multiauthored research approach that we will turn next.

Collaborators Collaborating

In putting collaboration into context, there is a further tier to consider, one that is rarely broached in anthropological accounts of research: the collaboration that goes on between ourselves as researchers. Working in teams made up of researchers with different levels of experience and disciplinary backgrounds has long been the norm in science research, but mainstream anthropology has until recently had a tradition of single authorship. In the changing climate of research funding and with a greater push toward large projects, this tradition is now challenged. The "community of practice" (Lave and Wenger 1991) is not such a familiar one for social anthropologists although applied medical anthropologists have long worked in medical research collaborations (for example see Anderson's 2008 account of the discovery of kuru, a protein-borne neurodegenerative disease in Papua New Guinea in 1960s).

For projects of the scale and ambition of the ISBC research, there was an assumption, at least on the part of funders, that we could easily realize the hoped-for synergies of collaboration. The question is thus not just How do we collaborate with "them"? but also How do we collaborate with each other? Our general assessment was that anthropologists are not particularly good exemplars of collaboration with one another (Elliott and Thomas 2017). This is not the place to account for the ups and down that we experienced as a team (and there were many). Rather, we want to signal the creative possibilities inherent in collaborative ethnography both as a practice and in writing.

Unlike the lone fieldworker producing an individually authored text, the ISBC research comprised a team who had to develop a collaborative practice. Given the foregoing discussion, it would seem disingenuous not to bring this perspective to the table. The ISBC project was an extremely large and complex research initiative. In its conception, it was far from conventional anthropological fieldwork. It was made up of a principal investigator (Marilyn Strathern), coinvestigators (Monica Konrad, Margaret Sleeboom-Faulkner, and Bob Simpson), research associates (Salla Sariola, Seyoung Hwang, and Birgit Buergi), and PhD students (Rachel Douglas-Jones and Achim Rosemann). The Durham team, who focused on Sri Lanka, comprised Bob, Salla, and Rachel—that is, a senior academic, a recently graduated PhD student as a postdoctoral researcher, and one student just starting doctoral research. Bob had worked in Sri Lanka over many years; he had begun working on issues related to Western biomedicine in 2000 with examining the reception of new reproductive and genetic technologies (Simpson 2004a, 2004b, 2004c, 2004d, 2007a, 2007b). This work put him in touch with many of the key people in the emerging field of bioethics with whom he was able to continue working throughout the ISBC research.

The prior and ongoing relationships that Bob had were crucial to the subsequent integration of the other ISBC researchers into the local networks. There was already a degree of trust and familiarity that made introductions to key people less of a challenge than they might have been otherwise (although this was not always the case!). Rachel, who studied the development of capacity building in ethics reviews in Sri Lanka, continued to follow her "object" by working in sites across South Asia and the Asia Pacific region. For her doctoral thesis, she produced an outstanding account of how bureaucratic standardization is made to engage with local ethical, political, and cultural norms and variations, and how, in turn, new standards emerge (Douglas-Jones 2012). Salla spent a year and a half in Sri Lanka immersing herself in the networks running clinical trials, including about four months observing each of the trials in hospitals, attending board meetings, visiting laboratories, and interviewing frontline researchers such as research assistants and investigators. During Bob's frequent visits to Sri Lanka, we interviewed ethics committee members, graduate students, pharmacists, technicians, auditors, and other key informants. The fieldwork on which this book is based thus spanned more than a decade. The relationships with our collaborators have continued through to the present day, and several of them read parts of the manuscript.

Over this period, we have been able to follow the fates and fortunes of the individuals, groups, and collaborative ventures in which they participated. Thanks to our relationships with the senior management involved in each of the trials that we observed, we had more or less unfettered access to the running of each of the studies. (*Nota bene:* It was not part of our research design to focus on the participants in the trials.) An important reason for the generous access we were granted was that in both organizations there was considerable interest in dialogue with social scientists about their work.

Our endeavor could thus be described as multipeopled. In a homage to the work of Marilyn Strathern, Adam Reed has taken up the question of how, in contrast to single-authored and individually owned marks of scholarship, we might properly acknowledge the efforts and inspirations of others. Reed prefers to describe the process as one of "blurred agency" (Reed 2011, 177). In our efforts to put this book together, we experienced a growing sense of blurred agency, encouraged by the time that we had spent together during the project: Bob came to Sri Lanka for Salla's longer periods of fieldwork, during which time we did fieldwork together, traveled around Sri Lanka visiting hospital sites together, conducted interviews together, and shared a house—which meant yet more long hours talking about our observations. During these discussions, we compared our observations and interpretations of what we had seen. Back in the United Kingdom, Salla was a regular visitor at the dinner table of Bob and Joanna (his partner), and we spent hundreds of hours talking and analyzing notes about the trials and the people involved. We drew mind-maps, categorized events, interview data, and observations, and looked for vignettes to capture the patterns we came across. As we wrote articles together and finally the present publication, drafts were sent back and forth, and there came a point when it was no longer clear whose idea was whose and who had written which parts. Our experiences had, to a significant degree, become merged.

Eventually, familiarity with one another's data, writing, and thinking meant that it became extremely difficult to draw distinctions for what could be individually authored. More to the point, it did not really matter—although we had different interpretations at times, these points of contention became part of the fabric of our analysis, which was multiple rather than aspiring to a singular view from nowhere. With that said, we have narrated most of this book as though from a third-person perspective. Thus, except when using direct quotes from Salla's fieldwork notes, our perspectives pass through one another, as do those of our interlocutors, in ways that minimize individual authorial ambition but hopefully set international research collaboration in a new light.

Collaboration as Method, Ethnography as Effect?

In this chapter thus far we have drawn attention to how our collaborative engagement with an epistemic community of biomedical researchers became mingled with the collaborative relations we were attempting to study. Inasmuch as we were studying the emergence and consolidation of collaborative research and bioethics in Sri Lanka, we were also engaging in discussions, participating in events, and leaving various traces of our own knowledge behind. All these activities fold into our overall intention to capture these worlds as an ethnographic account. Treating our own collaboration as an example of an international collaboration of the kind that we were studying is an example of how this reflexivity can contribute to an analysis of collaboration—we represented an experience of how international collaboration happens.

Ethnographic fieldwork is always an untidy tracking back and forth when it comes to the people whose worlds we are trying to make sense of. As such, our ethnographic contribution draws attention not so much to the difficulty of getting access but to the inevitability of being drawn into the assemblage of global biomedical science research. Yet too much involvement in the ethical and collaborative endeavors of the trialists ran the risk of our becoming advocates or apologists for the trials industry, or perhaps even being mercenaries of sorts. There were numerous occasions when we were introduced as bioethicists or experts in ethics—thus appearing to outside observers as investigators who were there to ensure that trials were conducted properly. People interpreted our research on trials, ethics, and collaboration as "quality control."

Although this sort of representation may be uncomfortable for an observing ethnographer, in the collaborative mode such labels by association may be difficult to avoid. Conversely, with too much detachment one will remain an alien—remote and peripheral from what is most meaningful in people's lives and daily practices. Too short a contact leaves the analysis shallow, and too much engagement risks the researcher losing perspective. Dealing with this oscillation in practice is both uncomfortable and demanding, as has been evident in the personal accounts of fieldwork going back to the inception of the discipline of anthropology (for example, see Hortense Powdermaker's 1966 classic *Stranger and Friend: The Way of an Anthropologist*). The language of relational engagement that anthropologists have devised reflects these ambiguities with some poignancy: "collaboration" (think *occupation?*), "complicity" (think *partnership in an evil action?*), and "para-site" (think *unwanted hanger-on?*). These are all terms likely to bring puzzlement and even alarm to those whose worlds we are trying to understand. Yet these are terms that were intended to dislodge an already deeply embedded conceptual inheritance that has structured the way relationships in research have been typically conceived: informant (think *police?*), field (think *boundaries* and *containment?*), gatekeeper (think *access* and *control?*).

Although it may be tempting to conceive of the anthropologist as entering, becoming immersed in, then exiting a "field," the dynamics, as we have shown, are rather more complex. The postulation of a field misses the point that collaboration is the dominant mode of knowledge production at large and anthropology is but one part of this. While collaborating, we were part of the agenda of our collaborators. Whether explicitly or not, we were seen as allies in the pursuit of strategic ends concerning the promotion of biomedical science and bioethics in Sri Lanka.

The process of thinking through issues of collaboration and ethics has been a long one, and it has been one where we have had a chance to reflect on collaboration as being not just about relationships that exist among "them" but also the relationship between "us" and "them"—and indeed the relationships among "us" as ethnographers amid the changing *mise-en-scène* of anthropological enquiry. Once situated in this relational web, it becomes increasingly difficult to separate the ethnographer from the fabric of the collaboration as it is realized in the networks, motivations, and histories of doctors, scientists, and policymakers working together. In this account, we have thus moved a long way from the idea that ethnography might be an appropriate method for gaining access to the work of scientists for studying collaboration. Indeed, collaboration itself becomes a methodology, with ethnography one of its effects. In the next two chapters, we describe the collaborations that were set up to enable two different kinds of trials to proceed. The first was an industry-funded trial of a drug to relieve joint pain; the second was a charitably funded trial of a drug to improve the survival rates of those who have ingested organophosphate poisons. Each of these examples provides us with a context to demonstrate ethnography as collaborative effect.

Chapter 3

THE JOINT PAIN TRIAL

Clinical research and clinical trials: Medical research studies designed to
answer scientific questions and to find better ways to prevent, detect or treat
disease. A large number of clinical trials are confined to testing the safety
and efficacy of new medicines.

(FROM THE GLOSSARY OF THE NUFFIELD COUNCIL ON
BIOETHICS REPORT 2002, 185)[1]

Ethics re-describes accountability as a matter of responsibility towards those
who will be affected by the outcome of certain actions.

(STRATHERN 2000, 292)

In recent years, the globalization of biomedical research has proceeded
apace. Commercially viable research that discovers and improves drugs,
therapies, and surgical techniques is no longer limited to economically
developed parts of the world but now figures in the national planning of
regions that are "economically developing" (Akrong, Horstman, and Arhinful 2014; Brown 2015; Chataway, Kale, and Wield 2007; Cooper 2011; Kamat 2014; Petryna 2009; Rosemann and Chaisinthop 2015; Sunder Rajan
2005; Zvonareva et al. 2015). A primary driver of this activity is to be found
in the commercial interests of the global pharmaceutical industry and its
quest for new research populations. Ever larger samples are required to
conduct statistically robust clinical trials, and the emerging economies of
the global south are attractive to the industry because their populations
are more accessible, cheaper, easier to manage, and comparatively "treatment naïve" (Cooper and Waldby 2014; Fisher 2009; Petryna 2009). Another significant pull factor from the developing world is the prospect of
shortening and reducing the cost of the drugs pipeline by relocating trials

activity to parts of the world where labor costs and raw materials are cheaper and the ethical overheads that attach to trials are lower than in the global north.

Expansion of trialing activity goes hand in hand with expanding markets for pharmaceuticals and the possibility of selling drugs to the billions of people in the emerging economies of countries such as Brazil, India, Indonesia, and the People's Republic of China. Across the economically developing world, millions of people are now entering a global marketplace as health consumers. Indeed, pharmaceuticalization has recently been identified as a natural successor to medicalization (Bell and Figert 2012; Dumit 2012; Sariola et al. 2015; Williams, Martin, and Gabe 2011). The term is meant to capture the pervasiveness of pharmaceuticals in the framing of health policy as well as the treatment of an ever-widening repertoire of conditions. The spread of pharmaceuticals to new markets in terms of their consumption and manufacture is closely linked to aspirations to participate in drug discovery and development. Yet in order to do this effectively, would-be sites of pharmaceutical testing need to anticipate and prepare in advance of any direct engagement with the global assemblage of pharmaceutical research. Anticipatory strategies include reassurances that the regulation, governance, personnel, and infrastructure are appropriate. If global industry standards such as those laid down by the U.S. Food and Drug Administration (FDA) and those found in guidelines such as the International Conference on Harmonization Good Clinical Practice Guidelines (ICH-GCP) are not met, there is little prospect that the international entourage of research and development will make its appearance.

When clinical trials began to expand to resource-poor regions, questions were raised about power differentials across regions and, consequently, the viability of international guidelines for ensuring the protection of research participants (Angell 1997). Doubts were also raised as to whether international ethics standards could be met in cultural and economic settings that were both different and underdeveloped. This was particularly the case in relation to the capacity for ethics review (Marshall 1992). Trials led by pharmaceutical companies in low-resource circumstances have thus long been criticized for undertaking research that is easily characterized as being extractive and exploitative (Kamat 2014; Sunder Rajan 2006).

To recognize and mitigate the power differentials in transnational research relationships, attempts to incorporate notions of social value, social justice, and benefit sharing have been made (Benatar 2002; Emanuel et al. 2004; Lairumbi et al. 2012; Njue et al. 2014; Zong 2008). Also present in these endeavors has been the notion of collaboration, which features as part of a strategy in which local researchers ideally engage as equals with their global partners in order to level what often appears to be a very uneven playing field (Emanuel et al. 2004). These concerns have led to a great deal of activity in developing-world contexts to ensure that structures are in place to review research commissioned by the international pharmaceutical companies considering running trials in low-resource settings.

One perspective that can get lost in the considerations of social justice and concerns over commercial research in low-income settings is that of local collaborators—that is, those who work assiduously to attract and host externally sponsored clinical trials (although see Petryna 2009 for useful examples from Brazil and Poland). In the trial that we describe in this chapter, perspectives of local collaborators are presented in detail in an attempt to illuminate the local interests, hopes, and aspirations as well as ethical apprehensions that arise when seeking to attract internationally sponsored clinical trials into new settings. Importantly, what our account shows is that the local researchers were not just reactive in the face of external interests but were highly active in creating and managing the conditions to enable the research to happen at all. They were interested in what collaboration could achieve more broadly. This was no simple working out of the hub-and-spoke model of research as development but evidence of bottom-up aspiration toward an alternative research future.

Converging Interests

The Joint Pain Trial, described in this chapter, was a randomized, placebo-controlled, double-blind, multicenter, phase 2 trial of a compound (which hereafter we will refer to as Compound X) for the relief of joint pain. The trial was conducted in a clinical trials group established in the Human Genetics Unit of the medical faculty of the University of Colombo and funded by an international pharmaceutical company. The trial aimed at gaining FDA approval for a drug that would most likely find its way into Western rather than Sri Lankan markets. Similar products were already available in international markets but not available in Sri Lanka.

Up until this point, there had been no trials of this importance carried out in the medical faculty. Consequently, the preparations to run the trial began many months before any recruitment of patients took place. For the trial to run at all, significant changes had to be made in both the infrastructure and the regulations for such research. With the cooperation of the trial team, Salla was able to follow the inception and workings of this trial. A clinical trial is a complex, multisite, socio-technical accomplishment, and inevitably any attempt at an ethnographic account will be partial and selective. Nonetheless, we were given generous access to the day-to-day running of the trial, and we have been able to produce an overview that captures how the complexity of trialing is accomplished in the Sri Lankan setting. This is a theme we return to in detail in chapter 6.

Numerous actors feature in the setting up and running of such a trial. In this particular instance, these included the sponsor's representatives, three senior doctors/researchers in Sri Lanka, four junior doctors who acted as research assistants in the trial, two pharmacists, a Sri Lankan ethics committee, and an independent monitor from an Indian contract research organization. Finally, there were the research participants themselves and their families and friends. The trial also featured a range of important non-human actors: the international policies, standard operating procedures, and guidelines that shaped the actions of the local trialists as well as the drugs, documents, and computers that gave the trial its material form.

The trial was funded by an international pharmaceutical company with offices in Australia, India, and the United States. As with the publicly funded trial we will be describing in chapter 4, the relationships that were formed in order to run this corporate-funded trial are an important detail in understanding how and why successful collaborations come about. The process was initiated by Sri Lankan researchers, who described how they were intent on bringing together the "right" group of people to collaborate to establish a clinical trials unit locally.

The project was initially conceived by an enthusiastic young professor from the medical faculty who had built up a strong reputation for hard work and leadership in a variety of fields in Sri Lankan medicine and health care. As a geneticist by training, his group's overall focus was on a broad spectrum of genetic conditions. His desire to advance the cause of Sri Lankan medicine had given him an interest in clinical trials as a potential bridge to international sources of knowledge, training, and finance. Bringing international clinical trials to Sri Lanka was part of a personal and professional strategy that closely mapped onto the country's scientific and economic development aspirations. As a first step toward the realization of international clinical trials on Sri Lankan soil, he established a relationship with a Sri Lankan émigré researcher working for a pharmaceutical company abroad. A few other trials had been carried out in the medical faculty previously, but the study being contemplated required more infrastructure than any that had preceded it. The attempt to engage with a global pharmaceutical company in the running of a trial locally was, at that time, hugely ambitious, and it brought with it much anxiety as well as excitement across the medical faculty—particularly for the team who would be running the trial. Much was at stake in terms of reputations and credibility.

Although the professor was the architect of the trial operations, he was not himself an expert in rheumatology. To complement the team, he therefore identified two arthritis specialists working in the National Hospital in Colombo. Neither of these doctors had conducted a phase 2 or 3 trial before, so a fourth clinical researcher who had past experience in clinical trials was also included in the team. The rheumatology unit had conducted a phase 4 trial (a so-called postmarketing trial) in the past, so this experience was flagged for the sponsors as an important piece of evidence for the group's claims of being able to successfully run trials to international standards. The doctors involved with the trial all had strong reputations locally; nonetheless, they had to convince an international audience of their credibility and credentials.

One of the striking features of the trial was the interdisciplinary nature of the group involved. Salla asked the professor about this and why he, a geneticist, was interested in running a trial on rheumatoid arthritis, which is not generally seen as a genetic disease. His response illustrated well the insertion of biomedical research into broader notions of development:

> I'm initiating this so that we can build expertise in doing clinical trials to help our patients who have genetic disorders. I have a plan to develop our unit to do more clinical trials in genetics. It's part of my bigger plan to become an international level research hub in several areas: clinical trials, bioethics, bioinformatics, genetics, and stem cell research.

With the objective of developing capacity on multiple fronts, the professor went on to explain how he got the trial team together and his longer-term vision for them. Assembling the group was one of the stages required in the longer process needed to set up an internationally competitive genetics group. It was his hope that, eventually, such a group would be able to attract research in areas more suited to their expertise to address the genetic problems facing Sri Lankan populations, not simply medical conditions of concern to the West that just happened to occur in South Asia as well.

This strategy signaled some important aspects of what has been simplistically referred to as "capacity building"—and along with it the range of motives that people have for engaging with pharmaceutical companies. However, to get to the stage where the group wanted to be, it was felt necessary to begin building an international profile by creating trial opportunities, even if these were outside their direct fields of expertise.

In the history of genetics, similar patterns have been evident whereby collaborations began with groups representing a range of expertise and interests in genetics before moving into the more specialized subfields that merely use genetics as a tool in their area of specialty. To build capacity in the other areas mentioned, the Colombo group developed collaborations in stem cell research with a group in India, in bioethics with colleagues in Norway and the United States—and also with ourselves, as a source of knowledge and expertise in research ethics. For the professor and his team, the trial was thus a vehicle to enable them to move forward on not just one front but several. The successful completion of this trial would enable them in the future to help patients with genetic disorders who might otherwise have little hope of relief in Sri Lanka, who could otherwise expect little by way of interest from researchers in the global north.

"Helping patients" was also identified as an important motivation for taking part in the trial by one of the two rheumatology doctors from whose clinic patients were recruited. For her, an important motivation for participating in the study as a researcher was the lack of access to new treatments in the Sri Lankan National Health Service faced by her patients who suffered from arthritis-related joint pain:

> I'm taking part in the trial for the patients, to give them access to new drugs, because so many of them are suffering. You would have seen them in the clinic, how many there are and that they are not really having any options. Nor-

mally, we pump them with steroids, and that isn't really good. This way the patients have at least more options. If it wasn't for trials, we wouldn't find new drugs. Ideally a trial should benefit your patients. This trial might not benefit the patients in the trial but might benefit others, and it would still be worth it. The ethics committee would have to decide on these things first. To make sure that they [the participants] aren't used as guinea pigs.

For the doctor, the ethics review was the mechanism to ensure that the intended trial would not cause harm to the participants—that is, they would not be used as the wrong kind of "guinea pigs." Appropriate use of ethics guidelines would, in fact, enable the researcher to turn an experimental compound into one that could legitimately help her suffering patients. She considered the risks of experimentation, when weighed against the status quo, to be worth taking. It is important to note here that despite Sri Lanka being something of an exemplar in terms of some health care outcomes in the developing world, access to drugs and medical services are still stretched. Sri Lankan hospitals are crowded, and access to drugs is often limited, especially those that are provided free through the National Health Service.

This is the context into which Compound X was introduced for trialing. Indeed, our study found that, as the doctor had noted, the ward from which the trial participants were recruited was bursting at the seams. There also was a large crowd of patients crammed into an open-air corridor who were waiting to see a doctor and get their medications.

What the patients normally would receive were drugs from the essential medicines list, a list of drugs manufactured by Indian or Sri Lankan generic drug companies that are intended to provide optimum cover for most diseases (see the discussion of the work of Senake Bibile in chapter 2). Many drugs are not on the list, however. These would be the drugs of highly specific efficacy—or, as would be most likely, they are simply too expensive for the system's overstretched medicines budget. Nor could such drugs be afforded by most patients should they choose to pay for them themselves. The situation that arises for doctors and potential trial participants alike is thus an "empty choice" (Kingori 2015).

Based on her fieldwork in Kenya, Patricia Kingori has argued that taking part in a trial under such conditions is not a free choice but rather a decision driven by the shortage of resources in government hospitals. These circumstances call into question the ideas of altruism and voluntariness in attempting to explain why people in such circumstances take part in trials. Melinda Cooper and Catherine Waldby (2014) have suggested that a more appropriate way of conceiving participation in these circumstances is in terms of clinical labor. In return for their "labor" in the trial, the patients are rewarded with drugs they might not otherwise be able to afford and a better quality of care and relief from some of the many irritations of a hospital visit, particularly the endless queuing and waiting.

In countries like Sri Lanka, the limited access that people have to drugs can prove to be something of an advantage when it comes to its suitability as a clinical trials site. Overuse of drugs is a common problem in economically developed settings, which makes the pharmaceutical naïveté and a lack of contamination by drugs in the developing world an attractive feature of the population. The clinical project manager for the international sponsor company, a native Sri Lankan who now resided abroad, was well aware of this fact, as he told Salla:

> Patients are available here. Elsewhere patients are often ineligible because they have had access to a particular type of drug, but here they aren't; it's a developing country, it would be too expensive. Only a handful of Indians and Sri Lankans can afford this. Thus, they are treatment-naïve. Other regions have been trialed to death, particularly in Eastern European countries where patient pool is small; even India is saturated. Elsewhere in Asia, medical practice is questionable, and we need to ensure we have good clinical practice. I am very impressed how things have gone so well and how people have been working together so seamlessly. More trials to Sri Lanka!

The clinical project manager here makes clear the longer-term aspirations that come with shifting trial operations to this new location and why Sri Lanka is a good site for carrying out trials.

Yet it is one thing to identify a country as having the right demographic profile and quite another to actually work there. As in the public health trial discussed in chapter 4, relationships, trust, and mutual confidence were key to the setting up and running this trial. The Sri Lankan team managed to persuade the sponsors and their agents that they could deliver an appropriate patient cohort and run a safe and successful clinical trial. Although access to patients and the patients' access to drugs were important factors in considering Sri Lanka as a study site, there were also factors that were specific to this particular network.

Confidence in the local team was reflected in the comments of a senior partner from the sponsor company who visited to fine-tune the reporting of side effects. While framing the company's interest in more commercial terms, he also endorsed the efforts of the local team:

> From a purely capitalist commercial perspective, the need for clinical trials has boomed for about fifteen to twenty years, and there is no halt in sight. From the third world perspective, the West wants drugs for their consumption; that's where the markets are. Regulation there is becoming more and more stringent, there is more documentation, ethical standards are higher, [and] regulation is stricter than twenty years ago. The second reason is that we were working with a guy from Sri Lanka. He said that he has contact with these people, they are all well-educated, they are all Western educated, and there is a good health care infrastructure and the patients need the therapy. He had all these connections. The professor came over to us and said: We are ready to do trials. So the major things for us were: one, access to patients, and two, having a good solid regulatory system. You want the regulation to work because of the high risk that is involved, so it's not just about obtaining good data, also you need to be stricter than what we'd normally do. These guys have ethical standards—they are basically U.K. standards. So for us, we went through the ethical guidelines and tick, they were great and the drug regulation was excellent. You don't just want an easy route through the back door. That's tempting but, well, unethical. From the corporate viewpoint, that's what's in it for us.

The senior partner in the company narrated a familiar story of why the global expansion of trials is taking place and just how the link via a Sri Lankan émigré working for the sponsor company had provided a crucial basis for securing the collaboration.

Significantly, it was not the weakness of regulatory mechanisms in Sri Lanka that proved attractive to the company, but their apparent robustness. The senior partner emphasized that the company was looking for places where there was already familiarity with international regulatory frameworks such as those operating in the United Kingdom and under the ICH-GCP guidelines—and, moreover, the ability to put these guidelines into practice. To make sure that this was the case, local researchers were offered further training on how to implement international standards. Having carefully reviewed the local provisions, the international sponsor company found the regulatory structures and operational practices available in Sri Lanka to be suitable and decided to go ahead. Having got to this stage, however, there was still a lot more work to do to get the trial environment up to standard.

Meeting International-Level Standards

Randomized controlled trials (RCTs) aim to produce replicable results. An important factor in ensuring that replication is valid are the conditions under which the data are created (taken up in detail in chapter 7). To ensure that results created at site A can be put together with those from site B, the conditions under which the trial is conducted must be made as close to one another as possible (Helgesson 2010; Timmermans and Berg 2003). When sites are distributed across research-rich and resource-poor settings, that challenge is considerable. In running the trial in Sri Lanka, it was important for both the local and international collaborators that there was harmonization with international standards, which required changes in procedure.

The first requirement in this regard was for the trial to gain ethics clearance from an appropriately constituted local ethics committee. The study protocol was submitted to the Colombo Medical Faculty Research Ethics Committee. In their assessment of the application, the committee provided the researchers with a list of concerns that they felt needed to be addressed before their approval could be given. These were as follows:

1. Enough facilities and rooms had to be provided for patients—a separate space from the "normal" patients to allow proper monitoring.
2. Approval would need to be obtained from the Clinical Trials Subcommittee of the Drug Regulatory Authority (DRA).
3. The researchers should not administer doses before DRA approval was obtained.
4. Researchers should clarify the follow-up procedures in case something untoward happened to the trial participants.

5. Data insurance arrangements needed to be clarified.
6. More information was needed on data and safety monitoring.
7. There needed to be a clearer statement as to the benefits to participants after the trial.
8. An ethics committee member should observe the taking of consent.
9. The sponsor–investigator relationship needed to be made clearer.
10. Publication plans needed to be spelled out.
11. Consent forms needed to be submitted in both Sinhala and Tamil.
12. The trial needed to be registered with the Sri Lankan Clinical Trials Database.
13. There needed to be oversight by the local hospital ethics committee.

What is significant about this list is its thoroughness and the fact that it went over and beyond what the international sponsors were expecting—for example, in asking observers to be present when consent was obtained and requiring registration on the Sri Lanka Clinical Trials Database. What these requests signaled, above all, was the seriousness with which the trial was being treated by the local ethics committee.

As this was the first trial of this scale ever done in the medical faculty, the ethics committee had heightened concerns about it. The professor in charge of submitting the study's ethics application and documents for ethical review described how at the meeting where the study was reviewed, the committee had given him "a hard time" and asked some tough questions about the trial: "My own people questioning me, it was really good. The committee questioned me regarding the cutting edge of the study. They didn't say: No, we don't want this trial to happen, but to make sure that we have [a] good job done of the review—valid, clear. They did not just give it to me because I'm a friend." Crucially, this was not just a signal to the researchers and their international sponsors about appropriate conduct but also to the local audiences—who might be suspicious of the engagement with an international pharmaceutical company—whose concerns the committee was not immune to. An indication of the extent to which the ethics committee was prepared to go in their scrutiny can be seen in their request that all informed consent procedures be witnessed by an independent observer that they, the committee, would supply. The requirement was that the observer should sit through all the consenting sessions, which exceeded the existing guidelines for recording informed consent.

By the next meeting of the ethics committee, the researchers were able to respond appropriately to all the demands made by the ethics committee. The trial was given approval to proceed.

The trial itself was organized across two sites: the hospital ward and a trial headquarters situated in the medical faculty, both of which had to be modified to accommodate the trial. The medical faculty buildings are located on Kynsey Road in Colombo, and they date back to the early part of the nineteenth century (the oldest being the Anatomy block, opened in 1913). The high-windowed, white-washed, box-like buildings were built by British colonial administrators to provide a home for the rapidly expanding medical education system that was then beginning to be run by local physicians and teachers. The buildings make up the four sides of a small courtyard, shaded by palms and now used as a car park. Although there was not a lot of room for on-site expansion for the trial, the high ceilings and generous allocation of floor space put in place by the original architects to ensure cool, airy working spaces allowed for ingenious uses of room dividers and mezzanines. The installation of air conditioning has meant that such spaces are not the dingy ovens that they were formerly; they are pleasant, cool, modern working spaces. As part of a general refurbishing of the building in which the Human Genetics Unit was housed, old spaces were reconfigured, and several new rooms were created. Old and dilapidated laboratories and stock rooms have given way to the well-equipped offices and meeting rooms in which the trial staff performed their data entry and other non-patient-related work.

Recruitment of patients was done from two busy rheumatology wards at the nearby hospital. In one of these, accommodation of the trial necessitated creating a space where participants could be screened in private, could be given the experimental compound, and could interact more informally with the research team. There were two connected rooms for this purpose, each about two by five meters in size, with direct access to a toilet. As part of the preparations for the trial, the walls were given a coat of turquoise emulsion and new wall fans were fitted in each room. One of the rooms served as a waiting-cum-social area; the other was the more private examination room. The social space had six metal chairs along the wall. The examination room had a bed with a plastic-covered mattress, one metal chair, a small desk with an office chair, and a filing cabinet. Although the setup was basic, the allocated consultation rooms contained all that was necessary to run the trial, including access to emergency facilities in the event of an adverse reaction.

The facilities were inspected and approved by the international sponsors of the trial; they were judged to be of appropriate standard for the trial to run.

All the changes we have described were necessary to run the trial. They show how it is not merely a trial's findings that are important but the material conditions under which the data were generated. Moreover, in carving changes into the physical space of a university department as well as the National Hospital, the trial also succeeded in creating more space and time for patients to experience care and attention, albeit in the form of monitoring for an RCT. Compared with the majority of the patients in the ward, the trial participants were clearly being seen in more comfortable conditions, and they experienced direct contact with specialist doctors. The adjustments made to the infrastructure would enable the trial to run in Colombo as it would have done anywhere else in the world—but in so doing it gave the Sri Lanka participants a different level of care and attention. This made the patients' decision about whether to participate something of an empty choice (Kingori 2015)—it would be hard not to agree to participate given these improvements over the status quo.

Recruitment and Consenting

A major concern for all those involved in the running of the trial was the business of informed consent. This crucial meeting point between local research participants and the global pharmaceutical industry in the guise of a clinical trial was one that was subject to close scrutiny by both the international monitors and the local ethics committee. Given what was riding on a successful outcome, the well-being of participants was seen as a central concern.

Each day, new patients were recruited by the two rheumatology doctors. Each potential participant was screened for the inclusion criteria, and their informed consent was recorded. Approximately 50 percent of the patients who were told about the research by their doctor came to hear more about the study and to see whether they fit the inclusion criteria.

In the trial rooms at the back of the ward, I [Salla] found four patients and their relatives with four junior doctors, [who were] collecting details about their medical histories and getting them ready to be told about the trial.

Shortly, we left for the senior doctor's/investigator's office to consent. We waited for him in a busy waiting room overlooking the medical staff handing over medications to those patients who had been queuing in the corridors for over an hour. Once the senior researcher finally arrived, we still could not start as one of the conditions of the ethics committee was to have an external observer present and this person had not arrived—we had to wait for longer. Phone calls enquiring where this person was ensued, and more waiting. Finally, she arrived, and we entered the senior investigator's office and got to sit in the large, air-conditioned office which was markedly calmer than the ward outside. The senior researcher greeted us good morning and began to explain the details of the consent form and information sheet. He explained the procedure of the study using words like "placebo" [and] "double-blind," at times using the English words. The word *"pariēshana"* [experiment/research] came out in every sentence.

On the days that Salla observed consenting, the length of time taken was variable. At its shortest, an explanation of the participant information sheet took fifteen minutes; at its longest, it took about forty-five minutes. In each case, the participants had been given the information sheets during a previous visit to the doctor, so they had been able to take them home and discuss them with their family. In most cases, the participants thus had at least a week to think about their decision and to consult more widely. As we demonstrate in chapter 5, these decisions were not so much autonomous (that is, taken by a single individual) as they were heteronomous, by which we mean taken in consultation with, and possibly with direction from, a host of others. However, in a few instances the participants were keen to demonstrate autonomy rather than accepting some degree of heteronomy. As one participant stated proudly, "I am doing this although my family is objecting."

In the lengthier meetings with doctors and participants, the list of topics covered included the objectives of the study; who the sponsor was, who had approved the trial, and what tests would be done; information on the length of trial, the randomization, placebo, and blinding processes, the possible side effects of the drug, the dosages, and the effect on other medicines; how to contact the team in an emergency, an explanation of voluntariness and the right to withdraw from the trial at any time; an explanation of anonymity; and information on the storage of samples, data security, coding, the benefits to participants, and compensation and insurance. However, when in a hurry, less time was spent going through the twenty-three pages of the consent form, especially regarding the long list of inclusion and exclusion criteria. What was never truncated, however, was the emphasis on the trial's experimental nature and risk. Patients were given the list of possible side effects, were told about the nature of randomization, and were informed about their right to withdraw at any time and who to contact should they wish to do this. As one of the doctors recruiting patients explained, "I think in this proposal there is a lot of emphasis on the fact that participants can walk out at any point. I emphasize that a lot, and it wouldn't change their care in this unit. I was amazed how patient-centered the trial was. Usually it is about the drugs, drugs, and drugs. Here, actually, I find myself thinking, 'How are my patients?' I wonder how they are doing." In the consent meetings, the participants and their families (who were often in attendance) were encouraged to ask questions, and invariably they did. They asked, for example, Can I take other drugs? I have a wedding coming up—is it possible to adjust the visits? Do we have to get admitted to the hospital? Can side effects occur afterward? If we get adverse events, will we get medicines?

Once these preliminaries were out of the way, participants were carefully weighed, measured, and sent to the trial room to continue with the health check questionnaires to ensure that they fit the inclusion criteria for the trial. In the trial room, the junior research doctors took blood samples, measured blood pressure, collected a detailed medical history, and enquired about past and current health concerns. As the participants made their way from stage to stage, there was a great deal of interaction among them along the way. They would peep at each other's questionnaires to make sure they were filling them in correctly, and they would confer with each other as to what particular questions meant and how they should answer them. During the initial sessions, some patients explained why they were interested in taking part in research. In most cases, relief from a chronic and painful disease was their main motivation for taking part. Many were extremely eager to take part, and on occasion patients cried after they were told that they did not fit the inclusion criteria.

Once the initial formalities had been completed and participation was confirmed, the participants would visit the "trial clinics," which took place each morning. At these sessions, they would receive the experimental drugs and undergo regular rounds of monitoring and measurement. For the doctors, these sessions had to be precisely timed, for example, to ensure that blood pressure was taken at the exact same time on each visit. However, this meant that the individual participants had time to sit around and chat with one another while they waited for their appointment. Indeed, over the weeks the participants in the trial got to know each other and developed relationships based on their shared circumstance. They were all living with a very painful condition, and being an experimental subject gave them common cause and a context in which to discuss it. As they shared their stories and experiences with one another, some concluding that they were being treated as "VIPs" (cf. Le Marcis 2015).

After the participants left the clinic, junior researchers continued doing paperwork. They tidied up the data that they had collected during the day, refilled all the forms, entered the data onto the computers, and filed the papers away. None of the richness of the day's encounters—the chat, the gifts of sweets, the stories of family problems and predicaments—made it into the patient records. (For a similar point about the work that goes into "cleaning up" data, see Biruk 2012.) These things were all an irrelevance and something of a distraction, but these interactions nonetheless became a vital lubricant that kept the machinery of the trial working.

For the junior doctors, the record keeping, data mounting, and associated paperwork were the heaviest aspect of their workload. It was a surprise to all the researchers that ICH-GCP guidelines were a lot more stringent than the ones that guided their "regular" academic clinical research, let alone their medical practices. As we see in more detail in chapter 6, throughout the trial the protocol had to be followed to the letter. The ICH-GCP guidelines were a new experience for everyone. The paperwork was audited on a fortnightly basis by external monitors, including the independent Indian clinical research organization who oversaw the trial process (see chapter 7). The auditor described his task as "to make sure that sites identify the correct patients, to ensure the safety of the patients, and deal with ethical issues or matters of confidentiality." Given the importance of the trial beyond the testing of this particular drug, the team of Sri Lankan trialists were anxious to do everything according to the requirements of the various assessors.

Success and Failure

As the Sri Lankan team saw it, the trial was their opportunity to prove that they could conduct clinical trials according to the standards of a high-profile international pharmaceutical company. As it turned out, the team were able to recruit their initial target of twenty patients very quickly. This early success led the funders to suggest increasing the number of recruits from the site to eighty. To make this happen, the group needed more staff, and they hired several additional junior researchers and another pharmacist.

The research continued apace until, part way through the trial, participant number 28 had what appeared to be a "serious adverse event." At this point the trial came to a halt. Three versions of why the trial stopped were in circulation among the researchers and the monitors. In one of the versions, it was the ethics committee who put a stop on the trial because of risks to the participating patients. A report was submitted to the ethics committee to say that the adverse event that triggered the concerns was, according to ICH-GCP parlance, serious but not unexpected—meaning that it was an event known to occur in this particular class of medicines (as distinct from a serious adverse event that might be unexpected, or grave). In another version of why the trials were halted, a representative of the pharmaceutical company explained how the ownership of the company changed, and they had lost interest in taking the research further. This was reportedly because the tested compound was a "me-too drug," meaning that the drug was not a novel experimental compound as such but a product for which similar versions were already in the market and in competition. In this version, the adverse event was incidental to the ending of the trial, which would have occurred anyway. In a third version, put forward by one of the coinvestigators, the trial did not stop by the command of the ethics committee; rather, after the adverse event, the study's data safety management board told them not to dose any new patients until they had reevaluated its safety, but those who were already receiving the drug carried on in the trial and were seen through to completion.

The adverse event had clearly dented what was otherwise proving to be a very successful trial. The literature on failure in science and technology makes an important point about versions of failure, suggesting that rather than seeing failure objectively, it is an illustrative point at which different investments are made visible (Kingori and Sariola 2015; Timmermans 2010). Rather than seeing failure in a positivist way as a negative finding or the inability to complete the trial according to its preliminary objectives, the team was anxious to demonstrate that the trial was in all other respects a success that gave them important experience of trialing in a global arena (a point we return to in the book's conclusion).

So despite coming to a halt when it was otherwise working well, the trial established a clear precedent for clinical trial activity at the unit. Among the positive outcomes recorded by the group conducting the Joint Pain Trial was the assembly of expertise to run trials in the future and a demonstration to an international audience of their capacity to do so. Crucial for the argument we are developing here, this was not only first-order development (for example, in physical infrastructure, personnel, and training) but also second-order development: competencies in the conceptual and epistemic discourses within which international collaborative research is framed. Indeed, after the ending of the trial, the members of the team set up a small, private, limited company called Lanka Trials.

Subsequently, Lanka Trials networked extensively, tried to engage new sponsors, and applied for ethics clearances for several new trials for over a year. However, despite the interest generated by the team, no new trials materialized; for this group the "rails of science" were not extended (Latour 1982, 155; Petty and Heimer 2011). Various factors made their progress difficult. In some instances, the ethics committee felt unable to approve the applications. In others, the team was not able to put in place an appropriate network of investigators. The final blow came with the global recession in the early 2010s, which saw a significant slowdown in international pharmaceutical trialing (Sariola et al. 2018). At this point, Lanka Trials disbanded.

As we show in chapters 5 and 6, this was far from the end of the story. Developments, epistemic and otherwise, continued across different areas of practice and personnel. Before considering these, however, we will discuss the second trial that we studied, the Paraquat Poisoning Trial. This trial is illuminating because, despite the similarities to the Joint Pain Trial in the scientific approach to RCTs, the collaborative ethos in the poisoning trial was significantly different, and important distinctions in trial practice and sociality begin to emerge.

Chapter 4

The Paraquat Poisoning Trial

In the side room of a conference venue in Chandigargh, India, eleven researchers from four different countries sat together with the intention of establishing whether the two research groups they represented—the first an international one based in Sri Lanka, the second based in India—could develop new research together. They were attending the 2008 annual international gathering of toxicology researchers. All those gathered in the room shared an interest in how poisons work on the human body and how they might be dealt with once ingested. Their shared hope was to augment and improve research into a pressing medical and public health problem in South Asia: the alarming numbers of people who die from ingesting pesticides (for example, see Patel et al. 2012 for an Indian perspective).

The Sri Lanka–based Australian director of the South Asian Clinical Toxicology Research Collaboration (SACTRC) had learned about the Chennai-based group through mutual research interests and contacts. At the Chandigargh meeting, Salla was present as an observer, and she recorded how the researchers set about figuring each other out and looking for common ground upon which they might, at some point in the future, start to work. They agreed they wanted to begin with something small to see whether they could work together around common interests and pooled resources. As the SACTRC director put it, "there is no point starting with something large like a multicenter trial to discover that things don't work out. That would be a waste of everybody's time." As we will see, the reference to "things" covers far more than just the science of clinical trialing; here, it encompasses the host of intangible qualities that people bring to their relationships, such as integrity, politeness, respect, and tolerance.

During the meeting it was mostly the Sri Lankan group members who asked questions: What facilities were there in Chennai? How were poisoning patients managed? What poisoning types did they have, and what had they taken? How far did their patients have to travel to the hospital, and how quickly could they get there after the poisoning? What research interests did the Chennai group have? Did they have ethics committees in place for regulating their research? The Indian group received quite a grilling, and after a long discussion a timeline was agreed on for the researchers to explore further the potential for working together. The prospects of a future collaboration looked good. Mutual research ideas were exchanged by e-mail afterward, and several months later a group from Sri Lanka went to visit Chennai to firm up the arrangements. Upon meeting and visiting the Indian partners, the director commented to Salla that they were "a goldmine." The Indian group had a functioning toxicology unit in a local hospital, their own poisoning ward, lots of patients, skilled staff, and good laboratory facilities.

In the encounter we have described, we might be reporting on nothing less than the birth of a collaboration—that is, the coming together of one group of researchers for a productive research engagement that could last many years. The shared concern with poisoning in the developing world gave an important *telos* or goal to their collaboration in the making. It not only provided them with a compelling justification for their meeting but also introduced a hoped-for mutuality. Given the seriousness of the issues at hand, the question was not so much: How could they collaborate? as it was: How could they not?

In recent years, there has been a move to bring biomedical research to bear on some of the developing world's most pressing problems. The extent to which biomedical research has failed to address these problems was highlighted by the Global Forum for Health Research when it drew attention to findings of the Commission on Health Research and Development (COHRED) produced in the 1990s. The COHRED report identified what it described as the "90/10 gap." Put simply, less than 10 percent of the spending on health research went toward dealing with the health needs of over 90 percent of the world's population. Since this startling statistic first gained currency, significant international efforts have been mobilized to address the health inequalities that it underscores. In recent times these endeavors have brought into sharper focus the diseases of poverty, such as tuberculosis, malaria, human immunodeficiency virus (also see Stevens 2004), and other less prominent or neglected diseases such as dengue and leishmaniasis, which blight the lives of many who live in low-income countries.

In commercial terms, these diseases have never been profitable to treat, so they have received little attention within mainstream biomedical research. The recent engagement with these and other problems endemic in the developing world has moved researchers beyond an earlier tradition of academic interest in tropical medicine and ushered in a broader interest in the inequalities of finance, gender, access to medicines, and the structural conditions under which diseases become "neglected" in the first place (Biehl and Petryna 2013; Farmer 1999, 2004; McGoey 2014).

These initiatives are currently subsumed under the broad heading of "global health," and they have opened a new field of interest and action. Initiatives such as the Global Vaccine Alliance, International AIDS Vaccine Initiative, STOP TB, and the Roll Back Malaria Fund have been established to target particular conditions. Funding for such initiatives has been provided by governments and international nongovernmental organizations (NGOs) such as the World Health Organization (WHO). Funding has also come from charitable and philanthropic sources such as the Bill and Melinda Gates Foundation and the Wellcome Trust. However, as one of the researchers in our study pointed out, these funders combine their philanthropic overtures with a research business model, which carries pressure to generate results and drive tangible change. Many of these initiatives have had the effect of blurring the boundaries that previously separated commercial, privately funded research and academic, publicly funded research. In short, there are few examples of either entirely publicly funded studies or entirely privately run research, as many developing-world research initiatives now combine elements of both. Clearly demarcated public–private partnerships such as the Medicines for Malaria Venture or the International AIDS Vaccine Initiative tend to operate with agendas that interweave commercial, industrial, humanitarian, nongovernmental, and governmental interests.

Increasing the amount and type of research performed in resource-poor settings has been one of the major objectives of COHRED and the subsequent attempts to help reduce the 90/10 gap (Haines, Kuruvilla, and Borchert 2004). In practice, a key mechanism to achieve this reduction has been the stimulation of international collaborations to address "local health needs" (Glickman et al. 2009; Mayhew et al. 2008; Simon et al. 2003). International collaboration in biomedical research is seen as a key opportunity for partnerships to develop that will bring about transfers of the knowledge, resources, and personnel needed to address gross inequalities in health research. It is within this broad program of action that the work of our second case study, SACTRC, might be situated.

The South Asian Clinical Toxicology Research Collaboration

SACTRC was established in 2004, a collaboration that grew out of less formalized cooperation going back to 1988 (Phillips et al. 1988). The research performed at that time resulted in publications that emphasized the particularly high suicide rate in Sri Lanka when compared with the region in general (see also Gunnell and Eddleston 2003; Ratnayeke 1996; Thalagala 2011). Out of these earlier forays into the causes and consequences of self-harm by poisoning, a network of researchers was formed that later became SACTRC.

The work of this group came to attention of Bob in 2003 when a scandal emerged in Sri Lanka amid allegations that a patient had died as a result of being in a clinical trial (see chapter 8; also see Simpson 2012). The case seemed to be particularly interesting as it brought into play a number of local groups with whom he was closely involved at the time. The impetus to follow up on this controversy in more detail became part of an application to the U.K.'s Economic and Social Research Council (ESRC), which eventually became the International Science and Bioethics Collaboration (ISBC) project. For the Sri Lankan element of this project, we were given access and full support for our work by the senior management of SACTRC. In 2008, Salla began a program of interviews and several months of observation in a hospital where several of SACTRC's clinical trials were being conducted. During the ISBC research (2007–2010), both Salla and Bob built close working relationships with people at different levels of the organization and have continued these relationships beyond the life of the original ISBC project.

The development of SACTRC began to be formalized in response to a grant call from the Wellcome Trust and the Australian National Health Medical Research Council. One of the aims of this call was to build research capacity in developing-world settings. The application was successful, and the network that was to become SACTRC was awarded a large program grant in 2004. Their objective was to build local capacity for handling poisoning admissions, and in so doing to reduce the high death rates from poisoning. The studies ranged from clinical trials to observational and pharmaco-kinetic studies. During Salla's fieldwork, the group had a head office in Peradeniya and were performing studies in six hospitals across Sri Lanka. The studies were run by principal investigators who were a mix of Sri Lankan, Australian, and British researchers and were linked to universities in each of these countries. The group had eight PhD students, some of whom were local and others who were part of the diaspora and returning after the war. There were also numerous managers, coordinators, and clinical research assistants (CRAs), all of whom were Sri Lankan.

The group was also supported by an international network of collabora-tors across South Asia and the globe. The phase 2 clinical trial on paraquat poisoning that Salla followed was funded in part by Syngenta, the company that produced the herbicide. Although Syngenta contributed to the funding, the researchers were anxious to point out that the company did not have any role in the way the research was conducted or the interpretation of its results. These factors combined to give the Paraquat Poisoning Trial a character very different from the Joint Pain Trial. In this chapter, we give greater ethno-graphic specificity to these differences as a prelude to our discussion in chap-ters 5, 6, and 7 of conceptual and epistemic shifts in research practice.

Hospital Relations and Frontline Researchers

Access to patients for the Paraquat Poisoning Trial was negotiated via con-sulting physicians in charge of the hospital wards where the poisoning pa-tients presented. To ease the way, senior researchers and principal investiga-tors would visit the hospital's senior staff to gain permission and establish good working relationships. At the time of our fieldwork, medical doctors

in Sri Lanka did not need to do research for their career to progress. However, due in part to the research-capacity building efforts of organizations
like SACTRC, this picture had begun to change, and more doctors are becoming actively engaged in research activities. At the time, this picture was
uneven: some doctors enthusiastically came forward as research partners, but
others kept their distance.

Crucially, in the Sri Lankan context, if the physician in charge of a hospital ward did not agree to allow work in his or her ward, it was impossible
for any trial work to proceed there. To recognize the considerable power
wielded by the physicians in charge is to enter the distinctive and consequen-
tial set of hierarchical arrangements that feature in Sri Lankan hospitals.
The following statement—in which a physician described his reservations
about allowing his patients to be included in a Paraquat Poisoning Trial and
why he subsequently changed his mind—shows how, in one instance, "access" to the patients in the ward was negotiated between researchers and the
consultant physicians.

> First, I didn't allow research in my ward. I didn't have exposure to trials al-
> though I would love to do them. The reason I didn't allow the trial was, one,
> I didn't think that the objectives of the study were valid. The argument was
> that with the lower solution of the pesticide there would be more survivors,
> and therefore more patients would occur who would need to prevent heart,
> lung, renal, and kidney failure. I didn't see this as a clinician. I felt that it was
> an unproven drug on anecdotal evidence. Second, proposing something like
> this would give the patients and the relatives unnecessary distress [by taking
> samples] and hope that they might survive. Third, I also thought that pre-
> interns [who acted as frontline researchers] are young and immature persons.
> Patients and bystanders are unable to understand randomization and might
> think it is unfair. I presented these thoughts to the senior researchers who ap-
> preciated my opinion. Then a couple of months later I saw the pre-interns
> going around the hospital and felt guilty. Was I hindering valuable research?
> I heard that a few patients had actually survived, and so I contacted the re-
> searchers to ask if I could still join and joined the contract.

Concern that he might be "hindering valuable research" changed this consultant physician's opinion on clinical trials on his ward, and his comments
signal important shifts in the way that a senior physician sees power and
dominion over the wards, staff, and patients. To allow "valuable research"

meant accepting the possible benefits not only to patients but also to staff. His change of mind suggests an important moment in the acceptance of research as a normative feature of life on a hospital ward.

However, although consultant physicians were the immediate point of entry in negotiating research access in hospitals, they were not the end of the story. The CRAs who served as the main trial workers were typically medical interns who had completed their basic medical training. Usually they were waiting to be allocated hospital placements that would carry them on into the next stage of their training. Because they were medically trained, they were more qualified than the fieldworkers working in comparable international collaborations elsewhere. For example, at many African global health research sites—and particularly in those performing observational and public health research—the workers collecting data are often lower ranking health care staff, non-medically trained volunteers, or individuals chosen for their supposed knowledge of the community that is being recruited (Kingori 2013; Sambakunsi et al. 2015). The CRAs in the poisoning trial had to work closely and carefully with ward doctors as well as the consulting physicians.

The consulting physicians visited the wards twice a day. Although they acted as the primary gatekeeper to the patients, each physician also had about six junior doctors working under her or him, with whom CRAs had also to maintain good working relationships. At the ward, the primary clinical responsibility for the patients was with these "house officers" (junior doctors) who spent most of the day in the wards. They diagnosed the patients' conditions, prescribed medicines, and followed the patients' recovery. In addition to the junior doctors, everyday care work was performed by nurses, who took blood, gave out medicines, put on bandages, and, most relevant to the poisoning patients, administered their gastric lavage on admission. There were also attendants who helped with the work of lifting patients, cleaning up after patients who had vomited or excreted, and assisted with the difficult business of administering lavage.

Given the number of personnel and the challenging tasks they faced, messages about research did not always travel effectively from the senior to junior levels. The incorporation of a new category of health care professional whose *raison d'être* was primarily to perform research rather than therapy was both novel and challenging. The negotiations and clarifications that followed the arrival of these new personnel on the ward often led to tensions.

The nature of these tensions was evident in a conflict that Salla witnessed between junior ward doctors and the frontline researchers or CRAs.

> Upon entering the ward, the doctors of the ward (five of them) were all at the doctors' table and started bombarding questions at the CRAs. "We don't know what you're doing to the patient, there are no documents, and we are responsible! Sir [the consulting physician] does not know either, and he will chase you out. You don't provide the patients with any counseling either! Is the paraquat test even valid? Only from the patient's 'bystander' [usually a relative] we got to know that you are giving some injections." The CRAs managed to hold their ground well, explaining that information about the trial should be in the patient's records and that even they did not know in which study arm each participant was. "You have to tell us what you're doing," the junior doctors insisted.

In this particular instance, the information about a patient's participation in the trial had gone missing from his notes—which were a bundle of papers and slips clipped together—and its absence raised suspicions among the junior doctors. They were afraid that something that they might subsequently be held responsible for was being done without their knowledge. The management of these relations defined the smoothness of the operations on a daily basis. A collegial and amicable relationship between the juniors was likely to result in a positive research climate in the ward and exchange of research findings. The CRAs, being the lowest in the pecking order, depended highly upon their confidence in conversing with those higher in the hierarchy and upon their clinical and research skills. An absence of communication could lead to situations like the one described here, where neither the senior researchers nor the consultant were available, which left the junior doctors and CRAs to sort things out as best they could.

At this point, questions of research ethics and governance seemed a long way off, and more prosaic issues of accountability and patient responsibility came to the fore. As many trial coordinators and CRAs were themselves quick to point out, grafting a trial onto the complex politics of day-to-day ward life might have begun with the agreement of the consulting physician, but it was likely to entail ongoing negotiations between junior doctors, CRAs, and other ward staff.

The CRAs, as we have already seen, were typically medical intern doctors using the year-long gap between the end of their studies and beginning of their placement as productively as possible. This hiatus in trainees' medical careers had arisen as a result of a backlog generated by the efforts to increase the number of doctors coming out of medical school. The need for a greater supply of medical students was in turn linked to the political conflicts of the early 1990s, which saw medical training disrupted due to the closure of many universities during the civil unrest and ongoing insurrection. Nowadays, the enforced gap year saw medical students keeping their hand in by gaining experience working as CRAs on clinical trials.

Although these interns were not fully qualified as doctors, CRA work gave them valuable experience and the opportunity to learn more about medical research. They were not in charge of patient care, but the CRA position meant that they could see research participant-patients on a daily basis in a hospital environment. Some of them even had the opportunity to carry out small observational studies for themselves. Their employment as research assistants in the toxicology collaboration usually lasted between six months and a year before they moved on to do their internships, after which they would go on to graduate as doctors.

From their position, the CRAs could explore the option of becoming a career researcher. However, research is not well recognized or supported as a career path in Sri Lanka, and there were strong pressures to pursue a more conventional career in medicine. The CRAs were also not quite so beholden to the senior researchers under whom they worked. Unlike junior doctors, if conflicts arose for CRAs they could leave without any great detriment to their career, if they wished. The repercussions for a junior doctor in a similar situation could result in a posting to an unfavorable location or the blocking of career progression.

In short, the CRAs were the key frontline researchers. They did most of the day-to-day data collection, and they were responsible for the negotiation of research ethics in practice. The CRAs worked either day or night shifts, with two CRAs working together during any shift. Where Salla did her fieldwork, there were six CRAs in total working on a three-week rotation: two people on a day shift, two on a night shift, and two on leave. During their shifts, they recruited new research participants, took them through consent procedures, and collected preliminary clinical data. In practice, the CRAs modified their version of the consent routine according to the patients' understanding of the research and depending on which study the patient was being recruited for. Often the dialogue would be short, with the CRAs explaining to the patient that what they had taken was toxic or lethal and simply asking for their agreement to participate in research. For this request, they would use the expression *"Kemathida?"* which translates as the rather passive "Do you like?" in the sense of "mind" or "accept" being involved in the research. (The recruitment procedures will be discussed in greater detail in chapter 7.)

The trainees who took on the CRA roles for the Paraquat Poisoning Trial were typically drawn from all over the island, and the work on the trial brought them together in lodgings. For many unmarried young people in Sri Lanka, living away from their parents like this is unheard of. Mindful of this fact and also keen to provide a sense of community for the CRAs, SACTRC paid for a house (which became known as the Study House) to provide a place where all the CRAs could live while on site. At the same time, the group lodging allowed the managers to help the CRAs in more pastoral ways and to have oversight of the CRA team. This work-focused domestic community had a mother figure in the form of a housemaid who cooked the meals and did household chores at the Study House. Despite the fact that young and unmarried men and women were cohabiting—an arrangement that normally would be frowned upon—the parents of the CRAs were prepared to allow this. They were confident that the young people were being supervised and that they were gaining good work experience and a salary that they would not otherwise have had.

Above the CRAs in the organizational hierarchy were the research coordinators. These individuals were mostly science or pharmacy graduates employed on longer-term contracts. Their role was to prepare the compounds to be tested, to perform the quality control monitoring of the data, and generally to oversee the work of the junior CRAs. Many of the coordinators described their employment and personal experience in very positive terms; they found themselves working in what they felt to be a good support network with opportunities to develop their own projects. In line with SACTRC's original capacity-building aspirations, the coordinators could also see future research possibilities emerging from their current employment in the form of further research work or study, either in Sri Lanka or abroad.

The research team had a small office near the hospital that served as their headquarters. From here, the CRAs would report for work and walk to the wards where the trials were being run. The wards were divided into men's and women's sections. If poisoning patients were brought to the hospital after

5:00 p.m., they were channeled to a receiving ward for preliminary assessment. If a longer stay was needed, they would be moved the next day to other wards. At night, the receiving ward became especially busy. There was a shortage of beds, which caused it to become overcrowded. At the entry to each ward, there was a book with the names of the people who were in the ward and their conditions, and it was from this book that the CRAs checked to see if any new poisoning patients had been admitted in their absence. There were usually between one and five new patients in each ward per day.

In this set up, the junior CRAs were quite clear about the purpose and objectives of the research they were undertaking, and they invariably expressed it in terms of helping patients. Moreover, they would link the idea of helping with the Hippocratic Oath that they would have recited as medical students, perhaps in their graduation ceremonies only months before. As we will explore in more detail in chapter 7, however, encountering the extreme suffering of patients who have ingested poison is extremely challenging. The vague exhortations to "do no harm" provided only the most general of ethical pointers when junior staff found themselves caught between a desperately ill person and their role as primary recruiters and monitors of subjects for a clinical trial.

In short, the CRAs found themselves in an ambiguous role. As researchers, they were primarily observers, but they would often find themselves witnessing distressing scenes and being beseeched by family members to actively intervene and help the patient. Helping was not their role—their priorities lay elsewhere—so scenes of CRAs offering whatever consolation and support they could to the families tended to take place when more senior researchers and management were not around.

Research as a Lifestyle

Among the SACTRC team were also a number of doctoral students engaged in hospital-based clinical research. The majority of these PhD students were either Sri Lankan or of Sri Lankan descent, and they were funded by the Australian National Medical Research Council/Wellcome Trust research-capacity building grant.

One of the doctoral students admitted that he knew nothing about research before joining the PhD program. He had graduated from medical school ahead of his cohort and then traveled around the world working as a doctor and surfing, his favorite sport. Although he was of Sri Lankan descent, he only knew the country from his parents' stories—they had fled to the United Kingdom and subsequently to New Zealand during the conflict that engulfed Sri Lanka in the 1980s. When the opportunity arose for him to do research in Sri Lanka, he saw it as an opportunity to learn about his roots while further developing his passion for medicine. He said, "In academia, doing a PhD is like a big intellectual thing, but in medicine you are seen as the . . ." He made a funny face and screwed his finger on his temple, indicating that it was seen as foolish for a host of reasons ranging from financial to ethical. "Why bother?" he continued. "You could have a good position, and drive a jeep. It's one thing to treat patients . . . [and another] to do research on them."

Many of the research staff were weighing the choice between a well-paid and respected medical practice and a research career that was likely to be uncertain and difficult. One PhD student described the engagement with research in biomedicine as a "lifestyle" rather than a job, conveying the way in which it demanded both a particular attitude and a consuming commitment:

> I could be earning a high salary at one of the private hospitals and not worrying about these things. I end up having to deal with a lot of the CRAs' concerns. One really needs to love doing research; otherwise, it is not worth it. I get whipped in the back by my superiors about my thesis; they are very thorough and ask for little, little details. It's a choice between having a lush lifestyle, or finishing articles in the evening. SACTRC is not a job, it's a lifestyle, and it is an ongoing thing; you're never quite out of work and out of the loop.

A third student, Sri Lankan by birth, went to complete his PhD in Australia and ended up staying there, returning to full-time medical practice. As Timmermans (2010) has described in the U.S. context, research provided a pathway for career advancement among the younger doctors. In the case of the Australian émigré, the benefits of local medical training were lost to Sri Lanka en route to employment in Australia.

For many, the choice of a not-so-lucrative, not-so-high status career was justified in terms of humanitarianism and a rhetoric of alleviating the suffering made all too visible in global health projects. One of the PhD students said that when he had first started research in Sri Lanka, he was struck by all the things that were wrong with medical services, ranging from malpractice to ethics: "You can't just be research-minded. For all the things wrong there is always something else that is worse. It is complicated to develop one area when others would remain in the state that they are. Can it be effective when other areas are so poor? But rather than critiquing, to change the system from outside, it should be worked from within." Pointing to the overall systemic structures, the experience of Sri Lankan hospitals led this student to make attempts to move beyond a simple scientific hypothesis and extend his research in novel, multidisciplinary directions that include policy, advocacy, and knowledge transfer structures.

For others, the challenging nature of the work translated into something akin to medical machismo. Working at the sharp end of global health inequalities was not just a humanitarian duty but also an adventure, which required one to be able to handle the "toughness" of the setup. Working in these settings not only imposed physical demands but also required emotional discipline. As one of the SACTRC principal investigators summed up the situation,

> Different individuals have different emotional approaches to the work that they do here. [PhD student X] really struggled here. He'd get really emotional and intense about all things that went wrong and say, "How can you just stand beside and look and not do anything?" [Researcher Y] had a bit of that as well, and he was very junior at the time . . . My take on this is that you can't get too involved, that is like the helicopter approach. You can't just save one and then go away; it's not a sustainable approach. I am very critical of "helicopter research." Some foreigner comes to have a bit of action and tell how things should be done and flies away. I think we think that if the project does not help people, there is no point doing it. Like in aid, giving money is not going to help them to improve medical care. I hate that missionary doctor approach. I believe in sustainable change; we can do that when you make a change in practice.

In settings where the local medical capacity is deficient, doing research can be seen as detached and frivolous, drawing the researchers away from the immediacy of administering help to distressed patients. But, as this researcher makes clear, being able to manage the feelings that such intense environments generate was part of the emotional work that their jobs required. Too much feeling and the researcher might become too involved with the immediate rather than the bigger picture—which in this case meant the promise of sustainable, evidence-based solutions.

However, despite the goals of capacity building, career development, and sustainable interventions that the collaborative approach created, the research funding cycle rendered their work precarious and unpredictable. The director of the group regularly bemoaned the "even bigger" picture in which they all worked. He said, "While creating capacity, the project may still be developing dependency on the international research circuit." The uncertainties and fluctuations of global research funding thus might lead to an inability to develop long-term strategies and continuity for the projects and staff. This precariousness meant that the researchers were always worried about their careers and prospects, and they often felt pressured to publish as a way of showing that they were achieving their targets.

In this section, we have introduced the organization SACTRC and discussed how, through international collaboration, it worked to introduce an ideology of research practice consistent with broader attempts to address global health inequalities. Achieving this aim involved a subtle blend of distance (from the immediacy and intensity of the presenting problems) and closeness to local context (to ensure that knowledge and skills were passed on and appropriately embedded in local practice). Here, the work of researchers from outside the country was to generate an infrastructure—material, social, and intellectual—that would direct the benefits of research into rather than out of the country. To get this formulation the wrong way around was to risk carrying out the aforementioned "helicopter research"—an unethical and unsustainable approach that would smack of neocolonialism.

However, an appropriate local infrastructure is but part of the story. In the next section, we turn to a closer consideration of the relations that made up the collaborative endeavor.

Trust

One question that Salla regularly put to the researchers was, What makes a good collaboration? The director of SACTRC answered the question in the following way: "I guess, firstly, some sort of agreed common purpose or goal among the people who are involved. It's certainly very important because I think it underpins one of the other things, which is that if you can agree on common purpose and goals then it's a lot easier to develop high levels of trust about what all the players' motives are." Significantly, in this view trust follows common purpose and not the other way around. This view was echoed by one of the SACTRC managers, who also placed clarity of purpose high on his list of explanatory variables: "You have to have a common goal and object. You have to identify the right people. Each member needs to have their task, their role in the project. Good communication needs to be the primary thing, and all things should be addressed up front. You need to find the right people who have the interest from our joint protocol, to give authorship acknowledgement and to work together." With clear purpose, the personnel and other aspects of the trial would fall into place. As the director also opined:

> To have a good collaboration you need to have a high level of trust, because in clinical research things happen. You can plan as much as you like, and you try to communicate things at various levels, but because of the complexity it's inevitable that there will be bumps. When you have those sorts of bumps you need to have trust so that you can have a situation where others can say, "Look, I'm pissed off." Everyone's trying to move ahead with the very best of intentions, and there has to be this common purpose, so you need that level of trust.

The clear-cut teleology of the trial, it would appear, was replaced by a rather more contingent working out of relationships, which fell back on trust and people's ability to suspend judgment and action long enough for alternative and perhaps more collaborative readings of other's behavior. In this respect, trust was seen as key to the social fabric that held the team together, particularly when difficulties were encountered.

Trust is what enabled allowances to be made and relationships to continue into the future despite what at any particular point might have seemed good reasons not to continue the relationship—what were referred to as the "bumps" in the road. In considering the work that the notion of trust does in relationships, as opposed to the more elementary question of what it is, Alberto Corsín Jiménez suggested that under conditions of doubt and anxiety, trust has come play the role of placeholder for robust knowledge, the knowledge based on the certainties of evidence, audit, and accountability (Corsín Jiménez 2011). Trust, he suggests, is an "engine of epistemic distance-compression: where knowledge, responsibility and mutuality collapse into an identical social form" (Corsín Jiménez 2011, 178). According to this metaphor, trust might serve as the "engine," and the "social form" that it drives looks very much like the collaborations that SACTRC was trying to establish.

However, what is of interest in the context of these collaborations is their international character. "International" here signals particular kinds of distance to be compressed—and very different readings of knowledge, mutuality, and responsibility come into play. Consequently, the bumps that threaten ongoing trust may be of rather different scale and form when working internationally and depending on where one is within the collaborative assemblage.

One of the areas in which we encountered frequent misreadings of collaborative intent was in relation to the management of hierarchy. In professional encounters, Sri Lankans are rarely expressive of their feelings. Confrontation is generally avoided, with conflicts sublimated and managed through compliance and passivity (for example, see Chapin 2014, 103). With these sensitivities in mind, good collaborations were seen as ones where a shared vision was underpinned by efforts to anticipate the local sensibilities. The ideology of collaboration as enshrined in earlier visions of the scientific norm was one in which there were ideals of openness and accessibility underwritten by presumptions of a flat and flexible community of co-working scientists. In Sri Lankan medical circles, on the other hand, relations are typically hierarchical and segmented, with high levels of loyalty presumed to exist between seniors and their junior staff.

Given such steep power gradients, confrontations were best avoided, and there was a good deal of compliance, even when juniors felt doubt or a lack of confidence in the actions of seniors. Suspicion and jealousy also are common, along with the idea that corruption is rife beyond the immediate world in which a person operates. Foreigners, in particular, are treated with caution. This is hardly surprising given that for most local doctors and administrators these international collaborations would often introduce levels of resources that could prove very disruptive when released into local organizational hierarchies.

Collaborations also take on organizational forms that local staff may find difficult to read. For example, SACTRC presented itself to local audiences as a "collaboration" rather than an institution, and, moreover, as one that eschewed hierarchy and presented itself as a loose confederation made up of little more than the relationships it comprised. This way of presenting SAC-TRC created problems for how power and authority were read. Against this backdrop, attempts by the SACTRC management to work in a spirit of open communication with local hierarchies could be a cause of confusion. For example, the junior and frontline researchers at times expressed unease at the lack of clarity regarding the structures, responsibilities, and authority in their work.

In institutional settings that are often conservative and bound by convention and protocol, this foregrounding of people and relationships rather than organizational form was troublingly radical. Thus, despite the attempts to establish flat and fuzzy ways of operating, the subtleties of working across divisions of labor were not without tensions and were apt to be reconfigured by local researchers into the more familiar hierarchal mode.

Authorship and Publication

A story related by the SACTRC director captures some of the sensitivities that underlay what, on the face of it, was a clearly defined and perfectly amicable relationship between a consultant and the research team. It concerned publication both as an index of efficacy of collaboration and as a marker of academic prestige. In an interview, he described the background to the misunderstanding:

> When we had a joint research meeting where we mostly discussed intervention type stuff, [we] asked if one of the consultants [physicians] was interested in interventional studies, and he said, "No, no, no." I said, "That's fine, it's good that we know you don't want to do that. You are in charge." The study that we did in his ward—with his blessing but not direct involvement—went on without him, findings were published, and he was acknowledged in the publications. But nonetheless really what evolved out of all of this was that he felt that we didn't value him and that we ignored him, and he felt that he had not been acknowledged enough. Part of this was because probably he had not even looked at the papers we'd sent him where we'd acknowledged him. Because of this, he decided to punish us. He was not going to allow any research in his ward at all; now he was really in charge. We spent a number of meetings trying to understand what the issue was. It took maybe seven or eight

months for him to finally come out and say what the issue for him was. I decided to write a short but simple letter to say that I was very distressed that he'd felt that he hadn't been acknowledged and to try and explain the process of research and that there weren't ten papers out of that research which he wasn't acknowledged in. There was only one, and he was acknowledged in it. Interestingly, a few days later he allowed us to come back into the fold.

This example illustrates similar issues about territories and power to those described earlier in relation to the physician uncertain about accepting CRAs onto his ward. Here, however, a misunderstanding about acknowledgment resulted in the closure of a trial site for several months. In a society that pays such careful attention to the observance of hierarchical etiquette, not being included as an author was taken as a significant rebuff.

Given the importance of patterns of authorship as providing "transactional traces of past collaborations" (Strathern 2012, 119) and the common desire to collaborate to gain access to publications, international opportunities, and recognition of one's work, the ward physician's response was hardly surprising. It suggests a pattern of sensibilities that do not match straightforwardly with those of the researchers. Publication was also an issue that frequently exercised members of SACTRC, as the director opined:

I think we try, when papers come out, to send copies to everyone who's been involved in the paper, whether that's an author or whether that's people who are acknowledged in the paper. When you're in the collaboration, you say, "Look, we're going to acknowledge the work you do." It depends on people's understanding of that. If they're co-authors on the paper, then they often know that the paper is in preparation. Normally you tell people that this is what we're doing. Everyone's work is acknowledged; these are authorship rules. If you want be involved as an author then there are certain things you have to do. People then have to understand that. Perhaps in the physician's view, acknowledgment was that he would like a silver plaque. Perhaps that's a good idea. People should have all got something they could stick up on the wall. That's a very Asian tradition. From an Australian perspective, I think it's very nice but unnecessary to have that level of acknowledgment. But at the end of the day if you've already got 130 publications it's not really an issue, but if you've got two, it is . . . I'm guessing on the spectrum of complete trust to complete suspicion, you know, probably a certificate would be very useful to make the relationship concrete.

The director's further reflections on the importance of acknowledgments and transparency in recognizing everybody's role in publication indicate the cultural mismatches that may occur in how acknowledgment is enacted.

The use of ghost writers in clinical research (Sismondo 2009) as well as the rejection of gift authorship has led the International Committee of Medical Journal Editors to draw up clear guidelines as to who should be acknowledged as an author. Including all who have contributed, ranging from junior and technical staff to project principal investigators, is an important objective of these guidelines. Those who have few papers and for whom building a curriculum vitae is crucial may feel upset if they feel that they are being used as facilitators and data collectors rather than being included as authors. Although this sort of critique was not directed at the international research in Sri Lanka, several researchers of Sri Lankan origin did mention that it was common in Sri Lankan academia at large for seniors to expect their juniors to do all the work—for which they rarely got credit. The importance of intellectual support from seniors was also underlined by another of the SACTRC managers:

> Publication is one of the main parameters of success [of the collaboration]. We have had about twenty to twenty-five papers each year. This year we've already had eight, last year we had eighteen. That's been a real success. Usually in Sri Lanka, supervisors take a long time to comment on papers and generally do not discuss things carefully to their students and provide intellectual support. Whereas, these supervisors make a change by putting their effort and sharing their experiences. Finally, we had funding flexibility and statistical support that allowed us to publish so much.

All the collaborators in SACTRC had agreed to work within accepted authorship rules, which included an early opportunity to be involved in research and papers in their area of interest. In the collaboration, authority was distributed based on effort, but there was also pressure to publish. Despite the collaboration being a nonprofit research body, its funders were seen to operate on a commercial output-driven logic of reward. Where publication and authorship were concerned, there were no discounts when it came to the demands of working in a low-resource, high-pressure setting. Those who in their role had found themselves spending a lot of time building the social infrastructure for the studies in the hospitals were at times criticized for their slow publication rate.

In sum, working to address global health inequalities through international collaborative ventures of the kind described here would appear to follow certain principles: sharing a vision, building on existing knowledge and experience, choosing partners with whom one can work, establishing clear roles and relationships, building trust and friendships, maintaining good commitment, and ensuring that collaborators are recognized in the outputs of the research. Yet the attempts to realize these principles by blending an open and democratic mode of working with local conditions presented some considerable challenges. We saw a wide spectrum of relations in play. These ranged from the thrill of working in difficult circumstances on mutually interesting and exciting research questions with companionate colleagues through to emotionally draining rounds of persuasion and diplomacy to ensure that access to the hospital wards was secured and maintained for the duration of a trial. Communication could easily falter, and mutual expectations would fail to be met.

The international and Sri Lankan collaborators were keenly aware of these difficulties, and they were perhaps unusual in the extent to which they incorporated an awareness of the issues into their practice. They were eager to challenge what they saw as the colonial legacy of tropical medicine, which cast the developing world as a place that is acted upon, rather than a place that performs the actions. Although they made an effort to eschew the hub–spoke, north–south, donor–recipient models of development by using collaborative work as their vehicle, the power relations still continued to be written into the modalities of collaboration in practice. Underlying the scientific aims of collaboration are a plethora of other assumptions, which may surface in day-to-day interactions. These interactions speak to the different scales of the research-as-development nexus, and they point to the importance of mundane, day-to-day relations in research practices. Here we see the importance of personal networking, securing employment for oneself and others, accessing training, and getting into positions to control the flow of resources to individuals and institutions.

The managers of the collaborations we studied were not unaware of these challenges, and they made attempts to rationalize them into short- and long-run strategies. Doing so required mindfulness of global research as part of a global assemblage of institutions and relevant research and health care practices as well as an ongoing evaluation of the relationship between local and international research cultures.

Collaboration in Practice and as Practice?

In this chapter and in chapter 3 we have provided a descriptive account of the running of two clinical trials. The trials we studied were both nested in socio-technical networks that used the same modality of knowledge production: randomizing a small number of patients as trial participants to see whether a particular drug worked. The trials shared a common methodology and scientific rationale, but we have shown how they were very different in terms of their purposes and the contexts in which they took place. They varied in the networks they tapped into locally and internationally, in who funded them and in what ways, in where they looked for ethics guidance and regulation, and in who they viewed as being the ultimate beneficiaries of the trials.

The poisoning trial was established with the aim of addressing a humanitarian crisis in Sri Lanka. It was broadly situated within concerns about the large discrepancies in health research funding directed at developing-world health problems, and it was initiated by international researchers with an interest in medicine in low-income settings. The research would generate important benefits in the form of academic publications and improved clinical guidelines for the treatment of poisoning admissions, which would help not only Sri Lanka but also other low-income countries facing similar problems.

The specific challenges for collaboration that the team members faced had to do with social relations and working within a hierarchical health care system that had limited experience with clinical trials research. To initiate and maintain the necessary social relationships required the cultivation of trust, particularly given that the motives of outsiders were apt to be viewed with suspicion. Differences in cultural background were flattened out by the emphasis on a common purpose in terms of the scientific enterprise, which was often expressed in sentiments such as "We're all scientists, and that's what counts—if we get along and you're good in what you do, we can collaborate." Ideally, the researchers gained no concessions for being from a "developing country"—science and its scientists would be as good as anywhere in the world, and science was presumed to be the medium they all had in common. In theory, this left no space for prejudices based on ethnic background, cultural traditions, or nationality. The ways in which the people who were involved in the collaborations talked about their groups suggested that it did not matter where someone was from so long as they wanted to work together, knew what they were doing, and got along well on an interpersonal level. These attitudes coincided with the research ethic that emphasized the broader benefits of the research and its broadly utilitarian purpose—seeking to gain the maximum value for the maximum number of people.

In the industry-sponsored trial, the dynamics were somewhat different. The initiative for developing the trial came from Sri Lankans, so the trial was embedded in local relationships in a very different way from the poisoning trial. In the industry-sponsored trial, the assimilation of international research into local medical settings appeared to be largely unproblematic. The researchers were working with the support of the established hierarchies rather than in opposition to them. As such, the financial means and mutual efforts were geared toward establishing an internationally recognized trial site that would thereby attract more international research. The research teams were intent on gaining experience with research ventures of the type approved by the U.S. Food and Drug Administration and to cultivate practical skills that would enable them to comply with the International Conference on Harmonization Good Clinical Practice Guidelines (ICH-GCP).

Performing trials at this level was used to show international and local onlookers that Sri Lanka was an attractive trial site from both operational and regulatory perspectives. This aspiration was realized by creating a distinctive space and time within the usual operations of a hectic public hospital ward. The pharmaceutical company's motivation for the Joint Pain Trial was, in the longer term, profit-oriented as the drug was intended for distribution in international markets. The drugs, if approved, would be too expensive for local consumers and would ultimately benefit patients in richer parts of the world. However, in line with the trialists' shorter-term intentions, the patients taking part in the trials derived immediate benefits from the study.

As in the poisoning trial, the relationships within the team were very relaxed, yet the functioning of the Joint Pain team was marked by adherence to roles and strict compliance with the protocol policed by outside agents. Local researchers were also mindful of structural imbalances between them and the international research community at large. They recognized the difficulties in raising levels of expertise in a context where first-class science education is in short supply, as are the resources needed to carry out world-class research. In other words, it was important for researchers not only to

advance the research but to work simultaneously to address deficits and imbalances along the way and collaboration was their pathway to this.

This strategy is consistent with our notion of first-order development described in the introduction—that is, one geared to setting up research units,
hiring and training staff, gaining high-impact attention, attracting further
funding, and improving the material settings of laboratories. The trial was
treated as a resource-rich stepping stone toward developing other types of scientific research and collaborations. Consistent with this more pragmatic approach to capacity building was an ethical logic that might best be described
as one of practical deontology—acting according to ethical expectations. In
this case, the expectations were dictated by the protocol and by the ICH-GCP
guidelines within which the protocol was framed.

In table 1, we summarize the similarities and differences between the two
trials. There were considerable differences between the contexts in which the
trials took place, but one common underlying feature for both was what one
of our interviewees referred to as the "developing country factor." Unlike research collaborations that take place in relatively affluent settings, those we
have considered here had to work against a backdrop of inadequate resources
and a vitiated health care system. Such inequalities posed challenging questions for collaboration in practice: Who controls the research agenda? How
can salary differentials between local and international researchers be rec-
onciled? How can the outcomes of research be rendered as local benefits
rather than only helping external others? Overcoming these challenges
was cited by researchers on both trials as practical and moral reasons for why

Table 1. Different features of the joint pain and paraquat trials

Features	Privately Funded	Publicly Funded
Knowledge	Proprietary	Humanitarian
Direction of knowledge	Out	In
Capacity-building aim	Build an international level group, enable further scientific research	Train local researchers and doctors
Regulation	GCP guidelines	Research ethics
Ethical logic	Deontology	Utilitarian
Marketing aim	Primarily Western	Sri Lankan/Asian

international collaboration was important. Collaboration was a means to gain access to international networks, publication outlets, and funding in the future. But above all collaboration established a viable, sustainable local research culture that could address local problems more directly and as part of a wider development agenda. These objectives, moreover, were strongly underscored by the local ethics committees. In short, our interviewees did not look on collaboration merely as a *practice* but also as a *value* (Strathern 2011). Moreover, collaboration carried potentiality: it was *strategic*, aspirational, and forward looking. Hence, the rhetoric of collaboration began to align closely with that of development, reflecting hopes for a future in which there would be progress and improvement.

This alignment might appear to be self-evident in its effects, but it depended in practice on a great deal of work on the part of the researchers to reshape their conceptual language and ensure that the categories were clear. Without this second-order epistemic work, transnational research would not be operable in the diverse settings in which it lands. In the next three chapters we turn to the question of second-order development and the ways in which the running of the Joint Pain Trial and the Paraquat Poisoning Trial introduced conceptual and epistemic changes in local practice.

Chapter 5

Localizing Ethics

The idea of the "human subject" as it figures in the guidelines regulating international clinical trials is a relatively new one in Sri Lanka and must take its place along with an existing repertoire of ideas relating to patients and the "sick" role. What does it mean, then, to render this concept operative in local settings as a necessary corollary of running a clinical trial to acceptable international standards? Here, we reflect on conversations we have had with those whose responsibility it was to answer this question. First, however, it is necessary to take a step back to consider how the idea of the human subject came about.

In the first volume of his *History of Sexuality*, Michel Foucault identified an important threshold in the transition to modernity in Europe, the point at which natural life began to be included in the mechanisms of state power—politics, in effect, gave way to "biopolitics" (Foucault 1978). Foucault argued that in the formation of modern nation states, control of people's bodies is key to their governance and a feature of this control is the delineation of subjects who are likely to think of themselves in terms that are individualistic, self-governing, choice making, and free. In this view, bodies take on a new importance as they become the sites at which state power is exerted in the form of regulation, measurement, and monitoring. Care of the body through biomedicine has emerged as one of the primary apparatuses to achieve this and out of which have emerged different modes of subjectification—that is, new ways of connecting an individual's interior states (subjectivity) with the external conditions under which they live.

In recent contributions to understanding the biopolitical consequences of modern biomedicine, a plethora of neologisms have been brought into play. These have included biological citizenship (Petryna 2005; Rose 2007), biomedical citizenship (Decoteau 2013), therapeutic citizenship (Nguyen 2005), pharmaceutical citizenship (Ecks 2005), and experimental subjectivity (Sunder Rajan 2005a). Each of these formulations seeks to capture the changing constellations of state, subjectivity, and biomedicine as these play out in a variety of different settings (see also Beisel 2015; Kelly 2015). These notions of biopolitics and governmentality and the insights they make possible are useful in that they enable us to map the different ways in which human life is rendered manageable as an object of expert knowledge and open to the legitimated intervention of the trialist.

The specific governmentalities that we are interested in tracking here are those that feature in the guidelines, declarations, and policies used to regulate clinical research globally. We also are interested in how these are made workable in local settings. The notion of the human subject as an entity that exists outside of time, culture, and place is found throughout documents such as the Nuremberg Code and the Belmont Report. These foundational documents have at their center the idea that the subjects of medical therapy or research should never again be reduced to a state of "bare life," as they were in the concentration camps of the Third Reich where they became "life that does not deserve to live" (Agamben 1998, 136). Ethics guidelines thus recognize research participants as agents who have rights to self-determination. The application of these rights is believed to shift power from the state to the individuals themselves, thus ensuring that people will not be exploited as part of medical research. References to the philosophical principles of autonomy and individuality reinforce this shift, and they are given practical instantiation through the process of ethics review. These are powerful precepts, but they are not without their critics. It has been argued that the philosophical underpinnings of bioethics are based on Western—even Anglo-American—rather than "universal" values (Durante 2009; Hedgecoe 2004; Marshall 1992; Turner 2003). This notion of the subject is fundamental to international policy documents on health and bioethics, but the idea of a subject that is universal, autonomous, and individualized is, while transhistorical and acultural in its utility, less convincing when carried into other settings (also see Holden and Demeritt 2008, 82).

Subjects do not exist in isolation. Recent anthropological theorizations of subjectivity have drawn attention to the ways in which it is always relational, porous, partial, discursive, and malleable (Biehl, Good, and Kleinman 2007). In this view, subjectivities are locally specific and situational, pointing to the need to understand context-specificities when analyzing the construct of the human subject. As Kaushik Sunder Rajan (2005) pointed out, subjectivity is not a "placeless" concept. Rather, we are dealing with particular regimes in particular places, and ethnography is crucial for capturing the messy, non-linear, and contingent realities that Sunder Rajan's observation implies (see, for instance, Das and Das 2007; Kleinman and Fitz-Henry 2007). Another way of thinking of subjectivity-in-context is with Michael Carrithers's insightful elaboration on the classic Marcel Mauss essay on the notions of *person* and *self* (Carrithers 1985; Mauss [1938] 1985).

In a carefully argued critique of Mauss, Carrithers interrogates the terms *person* and *self*—or, more precisely, the *personne* and the *moi*. The *moi* he describes as referring to conceptions of the self within a wider cosmos and as typically used to reference an inner life that is individualistic in its formation. Carrithers defines the *personne* as "the social and legal history of the individual in respect to society as a whole" (1985, 235). What is distinctive about this aspect of the person is the extent to which it reflects the "ordered collectivity" of which he or she is a member. In elaborating these concepts, Mauss was intent on making a specific point about the *moi*—namely, that it had appeared at a particular point in history. However, using textual evidence from fifth-century India, Carrithers demonstrated that this was not the case; he argued that it is difficult to divorce the outward looking, social individual from the inward looking, psychic individual in the ways that Mauss attempted in his essay. What began for Mauss as a simple Durkheimian oscillation between the individual and society begins to look like a much more complex dialogue between consciousness and history. In ethnographic terms, the relationship between *moi*-theories and *personne*-theories needs to be carefully specified if it is to be understood (Laidlaw 2014, 38–39). This distinction is important because it throws light on tensions that emerge regarding conceptualizations of the self as they are embedded in ethical guidelines and protocols. This distinction is not one of Western versus Eastern self but of the universal-subject-as-assumed-on-paper versus the messy, socially located, historical, contextual one found in practice (Simpson 2018).

This tension is elaborated by the social anthropologist Michael Lambek (2013), who has drawn attention to two kinds of personhood: the forensic and the mimetic. He traces the notion of the person as *forensic* back to the seventeenth-century English philosopher John Locke, who used this term to designate the temporally continuous and rationally accountable person. This is the "modern" person now written into legal documents, who is believed to be capable of making contracts that will endure through time and for which he or she will remain morally and legally accountable. Similar presumptions lie at the core of the "informed consent" procedures that feature in biomedical encounters, which are evident in the practices of signing, witnessing, and the retention of documents as evidence of informed consent. In these transactions, the forensic person is the one who is deemed capable of autonomous, intentional, self-originated decisions, who, as that same person, can appreciate the consequences of these decisions at subsequent points over time. Indeed, doubts about this particular competence provide grounds for overriding or reallocating authority to provide informed consent.

By contrast, Lambek introduces the idea of the *mimetic* person, a term intended to capture the routine and performative aspects of human social life that entail "embodied articulation unmediated by conscious reason" (Lambek 2013, 848). These are then not the rational and calculated acts necessary to realize informed consent but the messy entanglements that come with a quotidian ethics. In our everyday lives, we are multiple and shaped by our partial lives with others. These work at different scales; sometimes they might work together, and other times they may not. In the context we describe in this chapter, researchers who enact distinctively local medical practices when it comes to dealing with patients are also researchers within the episteme of global clinical trials. This is a juxtaposition that creates certain kinds of tension that require work and creativity to achieve workable resolutions. In short, in the constitution of persons, several dimensions— forensic *and* mimetic, continuous *and* discontinuous, conscious *and* embodied, fixed *and* malleable—are in play. Or, as Carrithers would have it, they are in conversation (1985, 255).

The account of this conversation that we develop here draws attention to the way that collaborations carry with them particular fragments of governmentality and imagined notions of human subjectivity. We show how these fragments, especially regarding the forensic person, become woven into a more extensive fabric of local history, politics, and culture that in turn shape local notions of subjectivity and personhood. Crucially, entanglements with these processes do not displace the existing modes of subjectification but are laid down as accretions upon those existing forms. In effect, in seeing research as development, what we are highlighting is the preexisting field of social "forces"—the power dynamics, discourses, and practices out of which the human subject is brought into existence as a *sine qua non* of international research collaboration.

The ethnographic entry into this field is not via patient subjectivity per se—we did not focus attention on research participants directly because the interest of our research was intentionally set at the level of collaborative strategies in international biomedical research. As such, we mostly worked with doctors and researchers as mediators of a kind who, in their roles as professionals, experts, and intellectuals, performed a crucial brokerage role in the reception of new forms of knowledge and the development possibilities that these enabled. Crucially, however, the researchers and doctors do not simply pass on such knowledge; rather, in the manner of the para-ethnographers and theorists of the human conditions they encounter, they also endorse, interpret, critique, and question according to the rationalities and pragmatics of their time and place (Boyer 2008; Holmes and Marcus 2005). In effect, theirs is a situated response to the essentialized, biologized, and individualistic model of the human subject that it was their job to usher in. We investigated the discourses regarding subjectivity and the human subject as they were emerging out of the engagement with clinical trials.

Among those we spoke to, it was clear that there were differing levels of exposure to bioethics and the new requirements for research governance. Some of those interviewed could be thought of as bioethics advocates and activists, who were very well versed in ideas of human subject protection; others, such as the junior doctors we described in chapter 3, had limited formal training in ethics. The answers of the latter to the questions put to them consistently returned to two mimetic themes or modalities that characterized their attempts to make sense of the idea of the research subject in the context of clinical trials in Sri Lanka.

The first modality concerned how their subjects were seen as family centered; that is, they were viewed not as autonomous or self-governing, as the presumptions of a Western-oriented bioethics would have it, but as heteronomous—that is, likely to seek the influence of others in their decision making. In the researcher–patient encounter, the subjects exercised a complex and blurred agency, from which others are not easily separated out.

The second modality concerned the centrality of medical paternalism in researcher–patient relations in Sri Lanka. Subjects are attributed with distinct forms of what we might think of as *patiency* (cf. Reader 2010)—the culturally specific ways of being a patient and with which goes a sense that, in this encounter, things will be done to them by doctors who are presumed to be benevolent.

Yet with new ways of imagining people's involvement in biomedical research, forensic personhood is brought to the fore. Correspondingly, but no less problematically for our interlocutors, the mimetic aspects of personhood must be suppressed. The result is an occidentalist discourse in which Western individualism is negatively contrasted with Asian sociocentricity (Buruma and Margalit 2005; Carrier 1995). As we will see, these usages are strategic, overly determined, and essentialized when deployed in the rhetorical play on what it is to be a person in Sri Lankan society. They are important when it comes to understanding the vernacularization of the notion of the human subject in clinical trials.

Family as a Decision-Making Unit

We now turn to an area of concern that surfaced in the accounts of many of the researchers with whom we spoke: the difficulty of squaring assumptions about the forensic, autonomous experimental subject with those of a less individuated, more specifically family-centered subject.

At a very general level, the researchers we interviewed all embraced individual informed consent as essential to the proper conduct of a clinical trial, a claim that was borne out in our own observations of the actual trial procedures. They explained that it is crucial that the patients are asked for their consent: "It is their right," one of the junior researchers proclaimed. However, they were also critical of the practical implementation of consent as typically enshrined in universal guidelines for human subject research (that is, seeking to obtain consent from an individual who is fully informed of just what the research will entail, what their rights are, and what the duties of the researchers are). The doctors and researchers were keen to point out that decision making in the context of medical research in Sri Lanka is not straightforwardly individualistic and autonomous, but family centered. A professor of pharmacology explained that in Sri Lanka, as elsewhere in Asia, it would be more suitable to think of the regional differences as what she described as "Asian bioethics" versus the more universal bioethical guidelines that she thought represented particular Anglo-American values: "I see the main difference in the idea of autonomy. First of all, Asian bioethics is more family centered. Ethics should be seen as responsibilities and duties toward others rather than as individual rights. The person should be perceived holistically in his or her context and life situation."

The professor implies that ethics—taken here as originating out of a Western philosophical tradition—are not value neutral; rather, they have key conceptual notions embedded within them. She sees the pronouncements of many Western bioethicists as based on individualism and individual rights. She presents a different vision of bioethics that, in her view, would be more useful in Sri Lanka than the version being ushered in via the international guidelines and capacity-building endeavors. She points to "autonomy" as fundamental to this tension and suggests that Sri Lankan culture is not individualistic—the subject needs to be understood within this context.

Yet what constitutes the boundaries of the context is fluid. All doctors who have studied at the postgraduate level in Sri Lanka were trained in the United Kingdom, United States, or Australia. There is no such thing as a "pure" Sri Lankan mindset. As one senior researcher commented,

Universal [bioethical] guidelines are not universal . . . The fundamental problem that I have with bioethics is that they are not centered on an Asian philosophical background and they are based on autonomy, which is a more of a Western concept. There is great room for thinking about this from an Asian, Buddhist standpoint. Of course, the problem is that we [doctors] are all Western educated and have adopted Western thinking. It is difficult to go back and study that. These kinds of ideas are not popularly [*sic*] discussed.

The target for critique in these enmeshed encounters is the notion of individualism, which is seen as somehow alien or antithetical to an Asian or specifically Buddhist viewpoint.

A poignant expression of the differing modes of decision making in Sri Lanka was given by a junior researcher working in the Joint Pain Trial: "In our culture anyone can't [= no one can] function as an individual. They [the participants] need their family support and to discuss all matters together at home with their families. Especially women feel the need to discuss with their families. They need their families' approval. Someone has to escort them to come to the trial." This response was given in the context of a discussion about consent, which had prompted the researcher to describe Sri Lankan society as family oriented. She suggests that decision making resides more naturally within a set of family relationships than as something an individual is expected to do. She also hints at the patriarchal nature of decision making in Sri Lankan families—women would usually be expected to turn to their husbands, fathers, brothers, or sons for advice. Moreover, this inclination comes from the researchers as well, not just the participants and their family members.

Forms of subjectivity that are not solipsistic but deeply rooted in others are ones that might grate with much of the thinking that informs an autonomy-focused bioethics. Yet among our Sri Lankan interlocutors they resonated strongly. They also figure in the long scholarly tradition in South Asian anthropology and sociology. In South Asia, the notion of a person has been described as *dividual*—that is, not individualistic but relational (Daniel 1984, 1989; Dumont 1970; Marriott 1976; Mines 1988; Trawick 1990). The term originated from McKim Marriot's discussion of exchanges of substance such as food and body fluids among Hindu families in India, suggesting that these substances render the boundaries that lead to the constitution of the individual as porous and partial. The argument suggests that there is an intercorporeality at work in these transactions that connects people in ways that are distinct and have implications for the experience of personhood.

Subsequent ethnographic studies have, however, suggested that the notion of dividuality has been overplayed (Jeffery and Jeffery 1996; Lamb 1997). In particular, the term has been associated with a problematic cultural dichotomy: *di*viduality describes a kind of personhood distinctive to South Asia that is set up in opposition to the much-vaunted *in*dividuality of the Western person. This is not a dichotomy that we want to extend here: all subjectivities are relational (see also Biehl, Good, and Kleinman 2007; Englund and Leach 2000).

Nonetheless, it is interesting to note that these earlier anthropological writings on dividuality echo the arguments made by researchers in Sri Lanka about the importance of others in general and in decision making in particular. Their arguments also resonate in accounts of what happens when forces push in the opposite direction—when people become cut off from their social networks. In Sri Lanka, there are widespread beliefs that there is vulnerability in isolation. This state is captured in the notion of *tanikama* (Sinhala) or *tanimai* (Tamil). These concepts refer to the sense of aloneness, loneliness, or isolation that people feel when they are cut off, either psychologically or physically, from others and most typically from their relatives. In this state, the sense of vulnerability people feel may result in illness or even a demonic attack, known as *tanikama dosa* in Sinhala (Daniel 1989; Kapferer 1983). Although the patients and research subjects were not described in terms of vulnerability, it was clear that researchers were quite comfortable with consultations in which multiple relatives were present.

The researchers were careful not to create situations in which their patients might feel socially and psychically isolated. A powerful illustration of this point might be taken from the way in which consultations with a patient often took place amid a small crowd of kin, all of whom listened intently and often offered their own contributions to what one might otherwise think of as a private communication. In other words, a particular model of sociality comes into play in the way Sri Lankan patients prefer to make decisions about their participation in medical treatment—or in clinical trials. It is an approach that typically incorporates others, specifically family members. What the researchers described is a process in which the particular notions of subjectivity that come with the ethics of human subject research appear to be at odds with the beliefs and values that they and their patients bring to these encounters. In effect, to create the autonomous, or forensic, subject entails stripping away social relations, rather than efforts to locate the subject within them.

The existence of these two discourses—an emphasis on individuality and autonomy versus relationality and heteronomy—within the clinical trial encounters left the doctors and researchers in a conceptual limbo. As we saw in chapter 3, consent often explicitly factored in the families of the research subjects. The subjects consenting for the Joint Pain Trial were sent away to give them time to discuss with their relatives what their participation in the trial entailed. As will become apparent, however, it is not only the relationship within the family that might influence the subjects' participation—the doctors and researchers see themselves as part of a relational process as well when they are recruiting patients to the trials.

Medical Paternalism and the Experimental Subject as Patient

Despite a barrage of new documentation and training—for example, in relation to International Conference on Harmonization Good Clinical Practice Guidelines (ICH-GCP) guidelines—older notions of medical ethics and the power relations between doctors and patients remain strong in the clinical trials encounter. For researchers in the Joint Pain Trial, for example, the conceptual leap between being "a patient" and "a research subject" was not an easy one for them to make; indeed, the research subjects were often spoken of as patients. The researchers themselves appeared to be perpetrating something of a therapeutic misconception in seeing their research subjects as recipients of certain therapeutic benefits from the trial, even when they were randomized (with some of them thus receiving a placebo).

Seeing research participants in this way locates both researcher and research subject in a familiar relationship. In this regard, all the researchers spoke about the inclination to medical paternalism, suggesting that the patients look up to doctors with great respect and veneration (for similar examples from elsewhere, see Chin 2002; Jansen and Wall 2009; Komrad 1983; Miller and Wertheimer 2007). A useful notion to introduce at this point is that of *care*, with a consideration of just what kinds of care the informed consent transaction might be signaling. We might begin with the distinction between "caring about" and "caring for." This distinction was elaborated in the context of organ donation in an essay by Sarah Atkinson (2016), who outlined acts of *caring for* as responses to known and proximate others, whereas *caring about* typically references concerns beyond the immediacy of everyday lives.[1] Put in Lambek's terms, where informed consent is concerned the doctors first signal that they are expected to care about the forensic person before they can begin to care for the mimetic person they have before them.

The researchers whose views we have considered here were concerned that in their world they might end up being drawn into *caring about*, when *car-*

ing for is what they feel they should be practicing as well as preaching. A senior researcher who was part of several clinical trials addressed the issue of medical paternalism:

> When conducting the trial, you read all the information to the patients, but the reality is different, and patients are likely not to understand any of this. [For example] You have a fifteen-year-old-boy and his illiterate father who have never been to Colombo and know nothing about clinical research. Is this really informed consent?! Patients here are complicit, and medicine is paternalistic. Also, patients here will be suspicious if you give them too much information. Patients will lose their trust in the doctor if you disclose too much. They think this doctor does not know what he is doing, and he will go to someone else who will take advantage of his compliancy. This is usually overlooked because you know that your intentions are good. But it's not about you knowing that you are ethical because it is easy to overlook your own actions if you are assessing yourself. Really you should have an external person to do that. With the backdrop of ignorance and paternalism, can we really use the same standards of ethics as in the West?

Like this researcher, many others also pointed out that the patients who were recruited for trials were predominantly from poor backgrounds (that is, they were attending government hospitals) and were uneducated, so they were often assumed to hold a mixture of allopathic and nonallopathic beliefs about health and the body. Given these assumptions, the senior researcher has captured the dilemma faced in inducting people into clinical trials when they have limited formal education and are deemed to have difficulty assessing the risks of their participation. Despite these shortcomings, informed consent was nonetheless seen by most of the researchers as a meaningful process. Moreover, putting patients through the informed consent process upheld the global ideal of individual autonomy, and they were also thought to be educated about this important aspect of Western medicine as a result. As such, the researchers believed that the patients they approached should make an informed decision about participation in a trial.

Even so, concerns remained about what to do when informed consent was compromised by the patient's inability to assess medical details; thus, attention turned to the question of responsibility. The senior researcher we interviewed did not argue for the creation of an (even more) enlightened patient;

on the contrary, the suggestion was that the attention should be given to the researcher as the person who is in control. Yet the self-governance advocated was viewed as problematic—there is always the possibility of misconduct. The researcher anticipated this criticism with the suggestion that monitoring should be done externally to avoid possible abuse of the patient.

Moreover, the researcher would appear to be suggesting that there is more to medical paternalism than just the patients' purported lack of knowledge about allopathic medicine and a simple emphasis on the traditional power and status of the researcher. The doctor–patient relationship is suggested to be a bond of trust, in which the doctors—should they live up to the ideal—look after their patients to the best of their knowledge. In the introduction of standardized clinical trials models to Sri Lanka, this aspect of the doctor–patient relationship was seen as particularly vulnerable. Another senior researcher (SR) describes how the conduct of clinical trials has come into conflict with the ideas of agency and patiency that underpin this notion medical paternalism:

> SR: What I feel is that going down this clinical trials route will generally contribute to further distancing the doctors from the patients. Our consent form generated such anxiety among the patients that I felt it was leading to distancing. There were instances where I had to talk to the patients for a few hours and then I thought to myself, What are you doing here? You've created so much doubt with the consent form in the patient. By pursuing more with the answers than they want probably to hear, I was contributing further to the distance. Patients are not looking at it from a philosophical viewpoint but the common propaganda. "Western pharmaceutical company is exploiting the Sri Lankans, or people from developing countries. Am I going to be a guinea pig in this trial?" So I thought to myself, This is not the way to get through to these people, there has to be another way. Informed consent as a tool isn't appropriate, but it is a standard. How do you get out of it?
>
> SR: What's the problem with the distancing?
>
> Medicine has become a financial transaction, and there is an aspect of profiteering at the expense of another. The context of clinical trials would fall into that. [The patient might think] What is there for him [the doctor] to offer this for me? In the phase 2 trial you don't really know if it works or not. Given that, when you tell the patient that this is situation, it raises the first doubt. "If that is the case, why does he want to give it to me?" Then various other constructs such as exploitation come in to mind . . . In medical pater-

nalism in the doctor–patient relationship the doctor knows best. And when the doctor knows what is best for me, why is he giving me this experimental drug? That's the conflict. That's why I feel that there has to be a better way of doing this. I just don't know what that is.

The researcher here is speculating on the fate of medical paternalism and trust in the context of clinical trials. In principle, by consenting to be part of a trial, the participants are asked to make a decision for themselves about participation. As another of the senior researchers commented, "You're a doctor, you're supposed to know what's best for the patients. If the doctor asks the patient too many questions [as when taking informed consent], the patient will think that that you're a bad doctor." This illustrates the interconnectedness of trust and professionalism: the researchers are expected to be in charge, and the process of consent suggests an inversion of the expected hierarchy, challenging the bonds of trust that are normally assumed to exist between physicians and their patients in Sri Lanka.

The direction of power and decision making is counterintuitive in the clinical trials setting when it is compared to the previous, expected situation of the doctor–patient relationship. Landing such trials in a context in which medical paternalism is the predominant ethos of doctor–patient relations, coupled with the limited knowledge of experimental research on the part of the patients, had given many of the researchers we interviewed cause for concern that their patients had agreed to be part of trials because they trusted the researchers' expertise in deciding what was best for their care—and that trials might even be part of that care. In this encounter, the participants were far removed from the model of the autonomous consent-giving subject who lies at the core of ethics guidelines and the ethics review process.

Although the patients and doctors were described as relating to each other on the basis of a (paternalistic) medical framework, the doctors and researchers we interviewed were nonetheless adamant that autonomy was crucial to the ethics of clinical trials—and, moreover, it was the ultimate right of the research participants. None of the researchers were willing to compromise the principle of autonomy and informed consent by favoring, for example, a blanket approval by an ethics committee. The researchers recognized that their patients have a lot of respect for them, and that their patients are often uneducated, with limited awareness of allopathic medicine. Thus, they claimed that they made considerable efforts to educate their patients so that they could make an informed decision about their participation.

Making Things Fit

In summary, the doctors and researchers described certain tensions when it came to reconciling the different kinds of subjects that appeared once they begin to introduce the experimental logic of the clinical trial. The human subject—implicit in the discourses of bioethics guidelines and fundamental to the effective conduct of clinical trials—appeared to throw into relief the preexisting relationalities in the doctor–patient-family relationship. This relationship began to be laden with contradictions regarding professionalism (how to be professional when being explicit and open marks one out as less than competent), paternalism (how to avoid paternalism when that is the very thing that many patients expect of a doctor), and the purported lack of participant knowledge and education (how to treat participants as capable of carrying certain information and making judgments when their competence to manage that information is in question). In effect, the clinical trials and the guidelines for human subject research within which they are expected to operate have begun to reorganize shared assumptions about agency and patiency in the clinical encounter. In effecting these negotiations and accommodations, the doctors, researchers, and ethics activists have played an important role as mediators who, by their creative interventions, make things fit. In chapter 6, we pursue this theme further by way of an ethnographic account of several episodes from the Joint Pain Trial.

Chapter 6

Negotiating Collaborative Research

In chapter 5, we described a series of tensions evident in the informed consent process and how doctors *qua* researchers managed these in an effort to realize research not simply as a biomedical advance but as a project linked to local material and conceptual development. Here we examine a further set of tensions that emerge in the conduct of clinical trials in settings where there is little by way of custom or practice to draw upon. We describe how in the Joint Pain Trial questions emerged concerning the normative dictates of research practice and the imperatives of medical care in the Sri Lankan setting.

As in the previous chapter, we show how ethical engagement emerges out of the research encounter rather simply being a set of values that are fed into it. The tension we set out to explore is captured well by one of the investigators who, when reflecting on the way that the notion of randomization is presented to participants, saw a problem, namely that all principles of scientific research needed to be conveyed first in order to put randomization in perspective. For him, the problem had two aspects. On the one hand, he described a gap in science literacy among the potential participants; to get them to perform as forensic, autonomous decision makers and to ensure that they did not mistake the trial for routine treatment and care, he had to explain about comparison and control in great detail. In other words, he had to make clear to them that randomization might mean they do not get to receive the experimental compound at all. He suggested that there was something profoundly novel about the way in which the experimental procedure and the modes of knowledge in which it is nested was configured in the local context.

As we will demonstrate, this researcher's insight proved to be telling regarding the ways in which clinical trials become embedded in the local context. As with the reflection of the idea of the human subject in the previous chapter, when we consider the standard tools of the trial—randomization, blinding, and recruitment—at the level of practice rather than prescription, the important role of initiative and creativity on the part of those running the trial becomes evident. First, however, we must look at what it was that the researchers were trying to accomplish.

Clinical Trials as a Gold Standard

Biomedical science derives much of its analytical and empirical power from the claims that are made regarding its universality. Irrespective of where the techniques and procedures for scientific experimentation are enacted, the facts that they yield should be essentially the same at any time, in any place. However, for this to be the case, much effort must go into the work of homogenization. Statistical categories, terminology, language, scales, measures, standards, and properties all have to be calibrated, demonstrated, and put into practice in order that they might become "immutable mobiles" of the kind Bruno Latour (1987) has elaborated upon—that is, things that might bring change without being changed in themselves. Without this work of standardization, the experimentation upon which development in biomedical science depends will not travel; even if it did, it would produce results that were neither valid nor transferable. So "when experiments travel," to use Adriana Petryna's phrase, a good deal of preparation must be done to locate biomedical research within the global scientific episteme (Petryna 2007a, 2007b, 2009). Typically, a large-scale clinical trial funnels standardized data from diverse settings into analyses that produce results that aspire to methodological plausibility and statistical robustness. Findings take on the character and currency of aggregated evidence, on the basis of which sound generalizations might be made.

The gold standard for clinical trials is the randomized controlled trial (RCT), in which subjects are allocated to different treatment groups under carefully monitored conditions so that the effects and efficacy might be evaluated (Timmermans and Berg 2003). Immutability and increasing mobility are guaranteed through ever more scrupulous adherence to the rules and procedures for clinical trials laid out in documents such as the International Conference on Harmonization Good Clinical Practice Guidelines (ICH-GCP). Evidence that these guidelines have been followed faithfully guarantees recognition and acceptance of the results by the wider scientific public, including drug regulatory bodies, academic peers, and journal audiences. Crucially, however, the demonstrable capacity to index local practice to global standards is for the consideration of national bodies such as the U.S. Food and Drug Administration (FDA), which grant licenses for new pharmaceutical products allowing companies to enter lucrative international markets.

The neatness of the RCT model and its claims to epistemic authority have been brought into question by a number of researchers interested in the processes rather than in the products of human experimentation (Cambrosio et al. 2006; Helgesson 2010; McGoey, Reiss, and Wahlberg 2011; Moreira and Will 2010). Here, the interest is in the mutability of mobiles rather than their apparent immutability. Paying attention to process rather than product reveals the modifications, negotiations, creative acts, and interpretations that underpin the successful accomplishment of a trial and how the "universalising rhetoric" of science operates in practice (Jasanoff 2005, 15). To borrow an analogy from Latour, those who are conducting clinical trials are not mere placeholders in the mobile (Latour 2005); rather, they are actors who follow scripts but also interpret and improvise their parts, drawing on a multiplicity of experiences, objects, and persons that are presented as unified, comprehensive experimental paradigms (Knorr-Cetina 1999).

With the arrival of clinical trials into new contexts, a key element is the tension that surrounds the new rules and practices that must be learned and the familiar routines that, as a consequence, must be put to one side. The disunity is not only based on technical abilities and competencies but also involves assimilation of different ways of thinking about how to read information from the bodies that find their way into the trial and how to act upon that information (cf. Adams et al. 2005). In conducting a trial, there are necessarily shifts in ideas about causality, induction, inference, and evidence as these typically operate in biomedical practice. There is no single specific tradition of thought nor one group of authoritative specialists; instead there is a kaleidoscope of hybrid forms, each with its distinctive character, that represent significant points of perturbation, negotiation, and accommodation in an otherwise smooth world of multisite clinical trials.

In drawing attention to "epistemic virtues," Lorraine Daston and Peter Galison (2007) highlight how persons who take on the role of knowers in these worlds are connected to the knowledge they produce, not only as practical orchestrators but also as its moral authors. Yet at the same time they must also strive to create knowledge in which the marks of the knower have been erased—that is, they aspire to gain "knowledge unmarked by prejudice or skill, fantasy or judgement, wishing or striving" (Daston and Galison 2007, 17; also see Zabusky 2000). Considering this apparent contradiction— between presence and nonpresence, seeing and not seeing, intervening and not intervening—requires us to engage not only with the products of science but with the social fields and cultural repertoires that inform the practices of scientists.

But how does research become marked with the "social" in a setting in which there is no established tradition of biomedical research by big pharmaceutical companies but rather one in which trialing and other large-scale science collaborations are only just beginning to take shape? This observation prompts a second question: in the work that is done to achieve universal standards in clinical practice and bioethical oversight, is there a single and shared conception of the social in play? As the previous chapters have suggested, the bringing together of scientific endeavors across large discrepancies of wealth and development suggests a number of warm themes: networks might be extended, knowledge passed on, good scientific practice disseminated, innovative synergies improved, a culture of technological dependence mitigated, subject protection improved, exploitation challenged, and so forth. With the arrival of RCTs, however, cool themes also arise, notably the ease with which collaboration and bioethics might help mask exploitation in settings that are resource-poor and inadequately regulated (these are discussed in more detail in chapter 8).

We suggest that as collaborations are forged, there is not merely a more socially inflected, interdisciplinary, multiauthored "mode 2" science taking place of the kind mapped out by Michael Gibbons and colleagues (Gibbons et al. 1994; Nowotny, Scott, and Gibbons 2001) but a more complex engagement between experimental practice and culture that might be better characterized as science practiced in mode 2^n, where the n counts for the multiplicity of negotiations that need to take place at the different sites in which the work of standardization is undertaken.

As described in chapter 2, the Joint Pain Trial, which was funded by a pharmaceutical company, was an early attempt by Sri Lankan doctors and scientists to participate in the global laboratory that RCTs have ushered in. To figure in this laboratory, it is essential that local practices meet global standards, and that this can be demonstrated, supported, and, most importantly, evidenced and audited. Like some landing strip for a latter-day cargo cult, the conditions for successful reception of this new form of wealth creation had to be built in anticipation.[1] Glossed as yet another form of capacity building, these activities include significant recruitment and training of personnel. This includes clinical research assistants (CRAs), trial managers, statisticians, and data managers as well as the formation of ethics review committees, the establishment of monitoring procedures, and the assembly of rooms, computers, and virtual networks that comprise the paraphernalia of the multicenter trial. Without this capacity, the benefits of future economic, intellectual, and social capital will not flow.

Within these networks, the RCT figures as a very powerful regime of knowledge making. The rigorous objectivity and detachment needed for the conduct of a large multisite RCT is capable of prizing apart other modes of connection that must be engaged with and rendered irrelevant to the pursuit of credible scientific evidence. As collaborators within this epistemic community, we were able to document the process of knowledge production and aspects of this reconfiguration: breaking connections, rupturing relationships, instilling a sense of detachment where before there might have been connection, relationships, and attachment as well as creating a complex assemblage in which existing systems, practices, relations, assumptions, and beliefs are transfigured to render the body an object of pure quantification. A mode of detachment that is inherent in the method of RCTs is introduced that operates on this messy reality and in so doing illuminates and thereby makes available for examination and modification practices that were previously likely to have been tacit. The crux of the argument we develop here is that in moving toward this detachment, aspects of existing medical and scientific practices must be disciplined and displaced. Erasing the knower from what it is that is eventually known is premised on the existence of certain kinds of knowers who must be trained and instructed not just in what to know, but how to know it; detachment of the social is necessarily preceded by the socialization of detachment. But what exactly are the practices that these novel forms of rationality discipline and displace?

To situate the findings, we remind readers of the Sri Lankan medical system which can be said to be a largely "craft"-oriented form of practice and one in which the full impact of an evidence-based medicine paradigm has not yet fully penetrated. As Stefan Timmermans and Marc Berg (2003) would have it, this is a system characterized by a "disciplinary" rather than a "mechanical" objectivity. Medical students encounter an authoritative approach in medical education and practice, with their relationships with established physicians marked by strong vertical hierarchies based on status, knowledge, charisma, and reputation. Relationships are marked by intellectual and professional patronage; they often follow lines of kinship, religion, class, and occasionally caste. Inasmuch as they are vertical, they are likely to be based on membership of a particular medical cohort or what might otherwise be thought of as the "batchmate" phenomenon. The steep power gradients that separate junior medical staff from their superiors manifest in a good deal of fear, concern to avoid offence, and a tendency to replicate rather than challenge received wisdom among the former. To fall afoul of a powerful senior is to risk long-lasting damage to reputation and future prospects, which are for many the primary pull of a career in medicine. The teacher's position in the hierarchy is in part based on managed ignorance—he or she keeps people in their place by determining what it is they get to know or are prevented from knowing (Dilley 2010; McGoey 2012).

When introducing RCTs into hospitals and clinics, one must engage with this existing "field of practice," to use Timothy Ingold's term (2001, 114; also see Bourdieu 1993). This is one that is marked by a developing rather than a developed research culture, in which there is an emphasis on medicine as healing, where relationships are highly stratified, and power differentials are vertical. In this encounter, a series of challenges emerge. These concern ambiguities regarding the roles and responsibilities in the conduct of a trial and include the place of professional experience in epistemology, the hierarchical distribution of knowledge, the nature of expert authority, the management of ignorance, the place of evidence-based medicine in a craft tradition, and ultimately the relationship between care and research in biomedical encounters (Davis, Hull, and Grady 2002; Mueller 1997).

In the sections that follow, we describe how, in the conduct of the Joint Pain Trial, the cultivation of detachment became central. We discuss how randomization, blinding, and responsibility for clinical decision making landed in a context where seeing, caring, and healing by the doctors prevailed. We conclude with a discussion about the kinds of changes RCTs bring to existing ideas of authority and expertise.

On Blindness and Vision in Biomedical Research in Sri Lanka

Once patients had been appropriately inducted into the Joint Pain Trial and their consent recorded, the next stage was the administering of drugs. Pharmacists prepared the experimental compounds that were supplied by the overseas trial sponsor, placing them in white boxes that had randomized number codes on them.

The story that we are about to relate took place on the day before the first participants were to be given either Compound X (the trial drug) or the placebo. In preparing to administer them to the research subjects, one of the research assistants noticed that something was wrong. The team of research assistants huddled together and studied the envelopes and the refrigerator where the drugs were kept, attempting to figure out what had gone wrong. They read over and over the randomization instructions that told them to match each kit number to the numbers found in the envelopes. Eventually they realized that they did not have the kit number to match the randomization numbers; instead they had been given information about which dose—active or placebo—each patient would be given. In effect, they had been "unblinded." This was a code break, and thus a protocol violation.

They went to talk to the senior researcher who was managing the trial. Lots of phone calls ensued, documents were written, forms were signed, and an anxious shifting of weight from one foot to another was noticeable among the assembled team as they considered what to do. They eventually concluded that they knew which doses patients 9 and 15 were going to receive. They reasoned that even if the remaining trial volunteers were going to be blinded according to plan, they could not unknow what these two participants were going to receive. As this extract from Salla's notes reveals, the senior researcher took charge of the crisis:

> They will have to randomize the whole thing again. "Call the patients and give them some excuse not to come tomorrow." He changed to Sinhala giving instructions. "We have to inform the patients, we have to contact these patients before tomorrow." In English, he continued, "At least now we know, we have got the experience." He picked up the phone to call [to the overseas sponsor], saying out loud . . . [as reassurance to the assembled group] . . . "It was not our fault. Not our fault, we were sent the wrong envelopes." Someone in the overseas headquarters picks up: "Hi, XX here. Listen, a small issue. You sent us the wrong envelopes. We have been unblinded, you need to re-randomize everything . . . Right, okay . . . I'll talk to you again in the evening." Addressing the group: "We will start next Monday instead."

At one level, the vignette describes an everyday episode in the course of a collective technical endeavor: a problem arises and is solved. The unintended deviation from what was planned has been diagnosed, the hierarchies are activated, the solutions are formulated, the judgments are made, and actions are taken—thus, the crisis passes. Likewise, the response to the crisis would not be much different in a laboratory or hospital ward anywhere in the world. At another level, however, the vignette gives an important insight into the distinctive work that goes into stabilizing the process of knowledge production in the Sri Lankan context and the importance of strategic ignorance (McGoey 2012). To explain this event, we will explore some local notions of vision and what these reveal about proximity and detachment.

The notion of blinding is central to the methodology of the clinical trial. Indeed, a representative of the pharmaceutical company emphasized this at every point: "Unblinding must be avoided at any cost!" Blinding is intended to avoid any possibility that those who are conducting the trial have any knowledge of which patient is getting what treatment to eliminate the possibility of bias on the part of the researchers as well as the patients. In keeping with the requirements of ICH-GCP, the documentation, including the patient information sheets for the trial, are translated into local languages. In this case, the languages are Sinhala and Tamil. The idea of double-blinding is hardly a straightforward concept in English, and it might itself require translation from the English of the clinical trial manual to an English that is more familiar to the layperson whose consent is to be rendered more "informed." The translation of double-blinding into Sinhala is little different. Put before a native Sinhala speaker with experience of translating documents from English into Sinhala, it was clear that many terms in the manual were not in common parlance nor easily grasped—they comprised neologisms, hybrid terms, and borrowings from English.

It is not our intention here to revisit a well-documented challenge in rendering science accessible across chasms of literacy of one kind or another. What is of note at this point is the glimpse that the act of translation gives us into some deeper epistemological issues surrounding the ways in which knowledge and its creation are perceived in different language worlds and how those worlds reflect the standardization performed in introducing RCTs into Sri Lanka.

We studied the contents of the consent forms and participant information sheets, translating and back translating them. In Sinhala, the term for blinding that was used in the participant information sheets and consent form was *ubhayā dṛśya næhæsumeṇ*—literally "double (both) vision negated." Interestingly, local medical translators did not use the colloquial word for blinding as the removal of sight (*andha karanava*); rather, the usage here refers to negated vision. Although connections between the idea of vision and the status of evidence are found in many different cultural contexts (Bloch 2008), consideration of the idea of vision negated, as distinct from the state of blindness, is subtle but important in a society in which vision and eyes carry a distinctive symbolic and metaphorical load. Vision in many South Asian traditions links to knowledge, realization, enlightenment, and indeed to animation and life itself—the Sanskrit root *drs* means not only to see but to behold, to visit, to learn, and to investigate. Someone who is enlightened would be someone who is educated, wise, and can "see." Blindness, on the other hand, can be a derogatory term that carries connotations of ignorance and darkness. In this sense, the vision that normally informs experimental research procedure meets an intention to prevent or impair it. Vision, something that is fundamentally important to human experience, is consciously uncoupled from its groundings in curiosity and empirical understanding. In the name of scientific rigor, blinding would render the doctor passively subordinate to scientific procedure, or at worst, uneducated, whereas negating vision implies an active impairment of a faculty that is otherwise seen as critical to medical procedures and experientially based knowledge. Instead, the Sinhala translation suggests an informed decision to look elsewhere for a moment.

The practice of "blinding" and randomization reveals a new kind of intentional unknowing, a mechanical or regulatory objectivity that had to be inculcated among the junior doctors dealing with the trial patients (Cambrosio et al. 2006; Timmermans and Berg 2003). Objectivity and the guarantee of scientific validity are achieved by eliminating certain kinds of relationships between the junior doctors and their patients; they are cut off from knowledge of which patients get the active dose or the placebo. Those who conduct the analysis of the data have no contact with the patients—they just compile the data. As far as RCT methodology goes, the researchers are ciphers in the conduct of the trial. Doctors who might otherwise follow their disposition as healers—that is, imitate the resourceful ingenuity of their teachers and invest emotional energy in the outcome of their interventions—must now practice a new kind of detachment. They are no longer operating in craft-mode but are recast as mechanical and meticulous monitors of the body and its functions.

The particular kind of detachment that is advocated here is primarily in conflict with the relationship that a doctor would normally have with a patient, the therapeutic relationship in which he or she would expect to exercise active decision making in the patient's interest. Especially in the absence of diagnostic devices or advanced technology, doctors typically have to decipher what the presenting problem may be by use of their intuition, experience, and logic, all of which are overruled by the epistemic requirements of the trial. The comment of the senior researcher made in the previous chapter is once again apt. The detached, blinded, conduct of clinical trials will result in "further distancing the doctors from the patients" and undermine the bond of trust between the patient and the doctor.

The clinical trials encounter results in an inversion of the power and trust relations that are expected in a medical context. Trust is replaced by a role in which the doctor is blinded: they are intentionally put in a position where they cannot influence who gets what drug. In the prevailing paternalistic relationship, doctors are expected to be dominant; the detachment that comes with blinding and consenting have the potential to undermine the mutual understandings of how a good doctor and a good patient should act toward one another. Eliminating one modality of attachment—to the patient as a person, to the idea of relief, and to the role of knowing intervenor—is intended to amplify others. Doctors become monitors of human subjects tuned to observe the precise impacts and "adverse events" of a drug that they may or may not have administered. Although the doctors now are detached, the Sinhala translation of blinding maintains that they are not ignorant or incompetent—they have simply had their vision averted.

The arrival of the RCTs introduced new modes of detachment not only into clinical relations with patients but also into relations among the medics themselves. Randomization, blinding, and responsibility for clinical decision making have been introduced into a context where men and women wearing white coats and carrying stethoscopes are associated with seeing, caring, and healing. These practices may have been tacit, but nonetheless they had to be challenged in order to produce the kind of data needed to meet pharmaceutical regulatory standards. The existing epistemic authorities and expertise were thus brought into question.

Changing Forms of Authority and Expertise

According to international standards, conducting a trial that had been unblinded would have constituted mismanagement and could have had a wide range of professional and economic consequences for everybody involved. As such, the episode reveals a series of dislocations that are interesting when set against the hierarchies that usually operate in medical settings.

Two things are of note. First, the junior doctors pointed out the error and brought it to the attention of the senior doctor; in the existing nonresearch clinical settings this would have been tantamount to a breach in etiquette. Second, the authority that was ultimately invoked came not only from outside the laboratory but outside the country—from the external monitors who instructed the team on the minutiae of data collection and the disembodied voice of the trial sponsor on another continent. Both these observations point to ways in which the novel rationalities that come with these trials unsettle the existing hierarchies and roles. The new forms of disconnection open up possibilities for challenge and critique that are not typically part of the relationship between juniors and seniors. The RCTs challenge the familiar, rigid, and carefully observed medical hierarchies, replacing them with one that is novel, diffuse, and emergent.

The contract research organization (CRO) monitor explained that his role was to report to the pharmaceutical company, although his organization was independent from them. Independent monitoring is required for trials that are aiming for licenses in international drug markets. In effect, the mediating role of the CRO—positioned between the trialists and the sponsor—is a lucrative insertion in the clinical trials assemblage. The CRO that was monitoring the trial in Sri Lanka had international offices in Australia, India, and New Zealand and had over 100 research sites across the world. For this particular trial the assigned monitor had a chemistry degree and was also enrolled for a PhD funded by the CRO. He visited the Sri Lankan site about once every two weeks, and he went over the conduct of the trial in considerable detail with the staff.

The CRO's role, as he saw it, was "to make sure that sites identify the correct patients, ensure the safety of the patients, and deal with ethical issues or matters of confidentiality." He had no contact with the patients but went over their paperwork—that is, he reviewed the patient case records and the informed consent forms to ensure that they were signed. He also checked that the patients were given appropriate time to decide and had had the details of their involvement explained to them. As he made clear, he was there to cross check and double-check the patient files relating to trial participation. If he found errors in a random sample of case reports, he would look deeper and try to identify whether the flaws were systematic, intentional, or unintended.

The monitor played a fundamental role in directing and correcting the trialists to ensure that the protocol was implemented in the same way across all sites. It was clear that staff were unfamiliar with and were occasionally annoyed by the CRO's attention to detail and the frequency of his questions. Things that were not normally documented had to be recorded according to the dictum "not documented equals not done." From the CRO's perspective, if test results, examinations, or the minutest of adverse reactions and observations were not recorded in writing then dated and signed, it was the same as if they had never happened. As he commented, "monitoring is not just about creating rules for the sake of rules according to guidelines but these are real questions regarding real patients." Interestingly, he also pointed out that there are no guidelines for monitoring, which seemed to be the only part in the standardized clinical research process that was not externally regulated and governed. This represented a loophole through which the inexorable involution of audit procedures might unfold in the quest for ever more perfect standardization. The insertion of the CRO into the clinical trials assemblage was thus not only lucrative but carried significant power when it came to disciplining local practices.

This level of detailed adherence to ICH-GCP guidelines was a new experience for the team in Sri Lanka, and they were surprised by higher levels of stringency compared with what they were used to in clinical research and practice. And these expectations ran through the entire process—from the pharmacists to the junior doctors up to the senior management. Observing one of the pharmacists preparing the drugs, Salla noted how carefully she did it, as if with respect: she put on her gloves, disinfected everything with alcohol, took a small box out of the cool box, shook the box ten times, removed four bottles from it, drew the content of each bottle into large syringes, then shook each syringe ten times. The content was then injected using a smaller needle. In between each action, she disinfected the workspace. Afterward, she put the needles into a disinfected plastic bag, then into a cold bag to be taken to the wards by a courier.

On the occasion that Salla walked along with the drugs to the hospital, the courier was the information technology technician for the group. At the hospital, one of the CRAs was talking to a patient—explaining the trial again while preparing to administer the drug and collecting medical history and further data. The doctor repeated that this was a phase 2 trial, and that the drug's safety was still under investigation. The junior doctors/CRAs were in charge of data collection from the patients, and they oversaw the injection of the trial drugs by nurses. With stopwatch precision, the junior doctors timed their questions for the participant. The junior doctors involved in the trial all said that keeping pace with the schedule of the protocol and the paperwork was the heaviest and most time-consuming part of their workload, and there was clearly a lot of it.

The importance of instilling the discipline of meticulous recording was expressed by junior and senior doctors alike. One senior researcher pointed out that everything had to be done according to the ICH-GCP guidelines:

> They want all information collected meticulously. So much detail! Sometimes what happens is that I work from 8 a.m. to 10 p.m. [with non-trial patients]

and sometimes I get tired and I cut corners and take symptoms according to what patients say rather than testing: "Doctor my shoulders hurt," and I'll just note it down. Here you can't do that. You have to test everything, and you can't use Tipp-Ex [correction fluid] with anything. Everything has to be recorded. Everything has to be watched very carefully. I changed my practice accordingly.

Another senior researcher pointed to the need to pay attention to detail and surpassing judgment about what detail was relevant:

GCP guidelines and their conduct was a new experience for me. Expectations had to be met with great attention to detail. Tons of documentation. They want it to be adhered to so carefully. Actually, it was very good. I didn't know if they were interested in something, whether it was trivial or not. Like when we were doing some blood samples after dosing, blood had to be taken every five minutes after. It is a protocol deviation if you didn't take it exactly at that time, and if you don't, then you have to inform the ethics committee.

This latter comment was revealing as to how the authority on what was "relevant" had been devolved.

In monitoring the work, a representative of the pharmaceutical company said that he had found some minor flaws in the way that the trial was performed. He thought that the local team was generally well-qualified for this kind of work, but he was concerned with minor faults in the documentation and with discrepancies in the dates and times—which were not seen as the fault of any particular coordinator but had arisen because they were doing things "for the first time." The point here, however, is not just the increased rigor in clinical conduct and audit but the doctors' responses to the expected paperwork, which reveal how the RCT changed the nature of what they were seeing in the process of gathering evidence.

The representative of the pharmaceutical company highlighted the tension further, when speaking about the trial team:

My duty is to follow the process, and I came here to guide these people, and this is said with all respect, these guys are great. There were a few things that needed talking over, and I preferred to talk things face to face. So I came to talk about [a] few things that were of major concern. It might feel like "oh my god," but then you remind yourself that these people are doing a trial for the first time and they can be simply discussed through. Some little things that needed guidance that helping through will improve.

Last time I came, I went through the files, and I noticed that there were hardly any adverse events reported. Reporting them is important, and reporting everything that the patients are telling so that the risk-benefit ratio is met. So in order to collect safety and efficacy data, I saw that hardly any adverse events were reported. That's very unlikely. If that's the case, you have a wonder drug! So you doubt that. Like normally in a period of four to six weeks you would have a number of little coughs and colds, some little things, you might cut your finger, whatever. All of those have to be reported as adverse events even if they don't seem immediately to be related. It could be that all of them are cutting their fingers while cutting onions and then when you're collating the data you think, "Hmm, maybe this has to do with coordination." So this morning I explained that.

Normally you'd see a lot more bad things happening, and it's hard to explain these things by e-mail or Skype or whatever, but I think it's best to talk about this face to face, so I hopped on the plane to come over.

The underreporting of adverse events led the company representative to speculate as to whether the doctors were making their own on-the-spot interpretations of just what might constitute a significant adverse event and were screening out much that might be of relevance.

The junior doctors who were collecting the data while working as CRAs were, in effect, doing what all their training had directed them to do—they were processing complex and diverse information into meaningful patterns, and deciphering diagnoses with limited testing facilities. Yet in the trial the intention was to suspend their diagnostic meaning making, to see all signs as potentially relevant. The significance would come later after all the data had been pooled, and it would be arrived at by statistical rather than experiential means. For the CRAs it thus seemed as though their usual abilities as trainee doctors were being replaced by a different set of competencies, which were largely determined by the dictates of the protocol and were carefully supervised by a variety of monitors, all of whom brought a different authority than that of the senior doctor or physician to whom the they usually deferred.

Old epistemic virtues and expertise thus appear to be displaced as the doctors began to think as researchers—and patients were reconstructed as human research subjects capable of yielding a wealth of quantifiable evidence.

From this perspective, the patient becomes a representation of sorts—a composite of measurements, readings, numbers, and other kinds of "evidence." Thus, in the quest for standardization, other stories must necessarily be overridden or lost within the logic of the trial. Knowing intuitively or tacitly—and connecting things up too soon—was one of the very things that could place the credibility of the trial in jeopardy.

Changing Practices of Knowing

With the arrival of the RCT to Sri Lanka, the merging and clashing of existing paradigms and new practices became evident: hierarchy met diffused power structures, craft-based medical practice met evidence-based research, and the doctors' roles as healers and providers of a utilitarian, benevolent service were overridden by the need for rigorously mechanical observers. We have presented RCTs as a distinct, powerful way of achieving a kind of "conquest of abundance" (Feyerabend 1999). Here the "tyranny of the particular" (Medawar 1967, cited in Feyerabend 1999), which must be overcome when setting up and running RCTs, is made up of existing modes of learning and practicing medicine. This includes local ideas about causality and inference in medical examination as well as the management of knowledge and ignorance in professional hierarchies. What the RCTs usher in are new ways of thinking about what is real and apparent, what counts as knowledge and opinion, what passes as objective and subjective data, and who has the capacity to make these judgments. Demonstrable induction into these ways of thinking and doing are essential if local experimentation is to have currency in the global scientific episteme of the multisite clinical trial.

W hat we have described are the ways in which doctors are, in a Foucauldian sense, "disciplined." They have been trained in an allopathic medical tradition, yet they practice in a South Asian setting and must necessarily bring themselves into line with the authority evident in the protocols and guidelines. In this, they are directed by the various monitors and managers who convey instructions from worlds outside the laboratory, the institution, and indeed the country. In submitting to these new authorities, the team began to think itself out of familiar biomedical routines, connections, and hierarchies and into novel practices of disconnection and detachment.

The process was one in which a great deal of negotiation, improvisation, and "bending" was needed to create the appearance of the standardized trial. This, we have suggested, might be thought of as not merely an aspect of mode 2 knowledge production but as mode 2^n, where n represents the cultural negotiations that feature as a crucial part of scientific activity in diverse country settings. However, this is not to imply that trials in Sri Lanka are in any sense run badly, deceptively, or inappropriately; rather, as we point out, in the running of any trial the "local" and the "tacit" are ever-present—and without their appropriate incorporation and management the new biomedical knowledge could not be created and put into wider circulation. More importantly, for an understanding of research as development, the material and conceptual benefits of international collaboration could not be fully realized in the local setting.

In chapter 7 we turn to a somewhat different example of the way in which the situated nature of the trial plays a part in shaping the way that bioethical considerations are worked out at the local level. We turn our attention to what happens when the mundane guidelines for the conduct of clinical trials are deployed in circumstances of extreme crisis. Under such conditions, there is of necessity a good deal of improvisation—or what we refer to as precarious ethics.

Chapter 7

Precarious Ethics

During the 1990s, Sri Lanka's tragic claim to fame was that the country had one of the highest rates of suicide in the world. This figure has been halved since then (Gunnell, Fernando, et al. 2007), but self-harm remains prevalent. The methods people select to harm themselves are varied but typically result in violent and painful deaths. One of the most common methods is by using drugs, toxic plants, or, by far the commonest method, the ingestion of agricultural chemicals (Eddleston, Eyer, and Worek 2005; Gunnell and Eddleston 2003; Gunnell, Fernando, et al. 2007). Pesticides and herbicides are easily available in Sri Lanka, with compounds such as paraquat causing a mortality rate of about 50 percent when ingested and others about 10 percent (Dawson and Buckley 2007; Eddleston, Eyer, and Worek 2005; Wilks et al. 2008). The pattern is replicated more widely across Asia, leading to an estimated 235,000 deaths annually (Gunnell, Eddleston, et al. 2007).

The link between these compounds and self-harm constitutes a serious public health problem in the region, but the issue is one that has until recently been largely ignored at both national and international levels. One way in which attention has been brought to focus on this problem has been through the growth of internationally funded clinical research and the development of evidence-based antidotes and treatment regimens. Although clinical researchers in Sri Lanka have begun to address the issue of poisoning in a systematic way, many patients still die as a result of lack of attention, inappropriate care, and a scarcity of drugs and antidotes.

We offer an account of human experimentation in a context very different from that described in the Joint Pain Trial. The trials described here focus on self-harm in rural areas rather than on pharmaceutical testing in an urban context within a research facility specifically set up for a trial. As described in chapter 3, the international collaboration team that undertook this research was not for profit and operated in resource-poor settings and on subjects whose economic, mental, and physical condition rendered them highly vulnerable. The particular kind of subject sought for these trials thus posed significant challenges for the ethics of human subject research. Along with emergencies, disasters, prisons, and other "states of exception," these conditions do not fit easily into the neat and tidy ethics of the research protocol but entail a contingent and negotiated ethics on the edge, a precarious ethics in which the researcher and the researched face critical situations and where time for elaborate exegesis and reflection is likely to be in short supply (see also Kilpatrick 2004). In keeping with this theme, it is not our intention to undertake an assessment of the use or feasibility of international ethics guidelines that proceed with an already clearly constituted and universal "human subject" in their sights. Rather, we set out to observe closely the conduct of the trial to gain insight into the way a rather different ethics emerged. We explored the movement back and forth between three positions that became apparent during research into clinical trials in Sri Lanka.

At one level, individuals admitted to the hospital who have poisoned themselves might be thought of as *abjects*—that is, they are stigmatized by actions that have placed them at the very limits of physical and social life. They have seriously harmed themselves in an act that often leads to death, marking the act as a suicide attempt. Julia Kristeva's formulation of the abject is helpful here (1982).[1] Having apparently rejected life but still living, the poisoning patient becomes radically excluded and pushed into a state of abjection. But this state of abjection is also the point at which they are recruited into trials, whereupon they become the *objects* of research and experimentation—they are available bodies that provide measurements, samples, and pathologies to be observed. However, becoming the object of research also opens up an expectation that they will be treated as a particular kind of *subject*, one to whom certain rights and protections apply as laid down in international guidelines for human subject research.

In the account that follows, the tensions that exist between the three positions are explored at the point when the poisoned individual is recruited into the clinical trial in a Sri Lankan hospital. This chapter is thus not about self-harm or suicide as such, or about the experiences of these patients and their families; rather it focuses on the ways in which humanitarian interventions, randomized controlled trials (RCTs), and human subject research are brought together in novel configurations and guided by an ethics that circumstances dictate is always going to be precarious. It is our contention that the configurations of abject, object, and subject found in our ethnography have important consequences for the recruitment of vulnerable subjects in a wide range of settings such as refugee camps, psychiatric hospitals, prisons, or circumstances of extreme deprivation.

In hospitals, other emergency admissions such as for acute myocardial infarction or accidents resemble the acute state of the poisoning patients, but they are not quite equivalent because of the stigma that is routinely attached to self-harm. The limited amounts of resources available in rural hospitals and the moral economy of resource allocation generate an additional layer of complexity for such admissions. Here, the inexorable logic of the trial and the morality of care meet in circumstances of dire emergency. We attempt to capture the kaleidoscope of definitions, assumptions, and constructions that revolve around the poisoning patient as the object of medical research. Each section begins with an excerpt from Salla's field notes and describes, as a continuous narrative, one suicide admission at a peripheral hospital. Each excerpt introduces a set of themes and a discussion of the complexities that underlie research into the plight of poisoning patients and their fate once admitted to hospital.

Suicide in Sri Lanka

I was visiting a hospital in North-Central province with Jagath, a senior toxicologist and a researcher at an international research center based in Sri

Lanka, to observe their conduct of trials. We got to the hospital at 9 a.m. The trial was managed within a general ward by junior research doctors who worked for the same collaboration as Jagath. At the hospital, the first thing we were told by these junior researchers was that there was a Paraquat—a weedicide poisoning case.

We rushed to the ward. The ward was very crowded—the space between the beds was less than a half a meter. There must have been about 40 patients in this ward in total; some shared beds, some slept on the floor. The ward was open on the sides but roofed, there were flies everywhere, and the sun was already soaring. Patients were shouting, moaning; some were lying quietly. We found the paraquat patient curled up on an iron bed on a plastic sheet, shivering. The patient was a twenty-nine-year-old man, brought to the hospital without relatives. He had long hair, beads around his neck, and wore a blue sarong. At this point, the patient was still able to talk and sat up at times looking around. When he looked around, his eyes were wandering, bloodshot, and wild. The paraquat patient had been admitted at 2.30 a.m. the night before. He had taken about 100 ml of paraquat, which is a lethal dose.

The man in the ward had deliberately swallowed a dose of a weedicide. The quantity was such that it gave him a very low chance of survival and would likely lead to rapid multi-organ failure and death. Paraquat, the poison swallowed, is commonly used in farming and [is] marketed as the most cost-effective product available. A significant downside of paraquat is that it is lethal when ingested by humans.

Many explanations have been put forward as to why the above scenario is currently so common in Sri Lanka. For some, suicide and self-harm have socioeconomic roots in the Green Revolution in which the use of cheap fertilizers, herbicides, and pesticides to enhance harvests were fundamental to achieving increased production and access to wider markets (for example, see Fortun 2001; Mohanty 2005). Unfortunately, these policies also increased uncertainty and debt for many farmers, which led R. S. Deshpande (2002) and B. B. Mohanty (2005) to describe these as "farmer suicides" following a "crisis of agriculture." In Sri Lanka, it has been claimed that after the country was opened to a market economy in 1977, the suicide rate increased sharply (Vidanapathirana 2007).

An alternative explanation to the debt theory is access to pesticides and herbicides—with the opening of the economy and the drive to increase production, more powerful pesticides and herbicides became available, making the likelihood of death from ingestion even more likely than before (Gunnell, Eddleston, et al. 2007; Manual et al. 2008). These claims are often based on evidence that is statistical in nature, which describes the incidence of suicide and poisoning across times and regions (see, for example, Gunnell, Eddleston, et al. 2007; Kearney and Miller 1985).

Psychologist-ethnographer Jeanne Marecek (1998, 2000, 2006) has sought to understand the meaning of suicide and self-harming behavior beyond statistical prevalence and basic socioeconomic conditions. She has pointed to the fact that suicide has an interpersonal component. People act out of anger, disappointment, and impulse. By hurting themselves, even to the point of death, they also demonstrate their pride or hurt to their family and friends while at the same time eliciting shame and regret (Marecek 2000, 2006). Following Marecek's work, Malathi de Alwis (2012) has argued that suicide/self-harm has become a normalized part of everyday experiences and relationships in Sri Lanka. (For a detailed description of the socio-affective states that lead to self-harm, see Widger 2012.) Insult, sleight, affront, argument, or being shamed in some way can result in what Jonathan Spencer has termed a "karmic entrapment" (1990). Relatives are made to suffer for the hurt they have caused, and theirs will be the awful karmic inheritance of having caused a loved one's death. The inclusion of others in acts of self-harm in Sri Lanka thus raises the possibility that in many cases the objective may not necessarily have been *self*-harm but a high-risk strategy to attract attention to personal distress (Widger 2012).

Yet another dimension is introduced in Spencer's anthropological work on violence in Sri Lanka, in which he argues that the high suicide rates have been fueled by several decades of political conflict, communal violence, and a high number of homicides, which have routinized violence of all kinds, including self-harm (Spencer 1990). In similar vein, Waltraud Bolz (2002) links the political conflict in which the island has been engulfed with individual experiences, arguing that suicide is caused by a lack of conflict-resolution skills in the face of repressive religion, pressure to respect authority, and periods of violent conflict. She argues that people have few means to deal with confrontation other than through violence, be it toward self or others (Bolz 2002). These arguments would suggest that self-harm is symptomatic of a desensitization to violence in a society that has been struggling with major political upheavals for the past thirty years. (But for an alternative view on the role of war and other political upheavals in suicide, see Gunnell, Eddleston, et al. 2007; Widger 2012.)

The literature often talks about suicide and self-harm interchangeably, as it is unclear whether the person actually intended to die. In fact, some authors prefer to speak only about self-harm rather than suicide, arguing that very few of the people who have taken poison or burned themselves (a second preferred method of self-harm in rural settings) actually wanted to die (Konradsen, Hoek, and Peiris 2006; Laloe and Ganesan 2002). Epidemiological evidence produced by the toxicologists and public health researchers working in this field point to the availability of a new generation of even more powerful pesticides that are both freely available and more lethal as a major factor in making acts of self-harm likely to result in death (Gunnell, Fernando, et al. 2007). These numbers have shifted the problem from being one of tragic individual acts to the level of population, epidemiology, and national policy.

Perceiving suicide as self-harm that unfortunately results in death has opened up public health discussions about social and medical policies that ought to be in place to reduce the suffering and death that follows self-harm (Pearson et al. 2015; Ratnayeke 1996). A presidential commission of inquiry in 1995 brought this problem to the fore and led to changes in policy. Subsequently, suicide was decriminalized (De Alwis 2012), and attention was given to policies to tackle the different ways in which suicide is attempted. Notable among these were the efforts to reduce the availability of lethal substances. Tackling the methods available for self-harm helped to bring to light assumptions about the cultural embeddedness of suicidal ideation and action. Here the public health problem had to do with the toxicity of agrochemicals and health and safety standards rather than a "cultural fact" that Sri Lankans are simply prone to commit suicide. Over the course of our fieldwork, examples of the policies identified to deal with poisoning included smaller packaging sizes, control over sales, increased taxation, warnings on the packaging to suggest that ingesting pesticides and herbicides is harmful, and banning of the most harmful pesticides.

Whatever the reasons for suicide and self-harm, the fact is that hundreds of men, women, and young people are admitted to hospitals after having harmed themselves using a variety of methods. In Sri Lanka, there is a profound ambivalence toward those who attempt suicide, not least because they have broken a prohibition on taking life that is fundamental to Buddhist, Muslim, and Christian beliefs. Those who survive the initial attempt are typically admitted to the nearest hospital by an entourage of distraught relatives and neighbors. In rural areas, the admission might follow a long journey along poor roads in a lorry, taxi, or three-wheeler. At the hospital, the suicide patients are often stigmatized for their actions. The barely alive patient admitted to the hospital after having taken poison has rendered himself or herself an abject—someone who has sunk into a state of hopelessness, distress, and desperation.

At the Hospital

A test was done to confirm that the poison that the male patient had taken was indeed paraquat—one of the most lethal ones—and it came out positive. Since being admitted, he had not received any care from the nurses and doctors in the ward. Upon arrival, he had been under the influence of alcohol and quite drunk. Jagath said that he should have been put on a drip straight-away to give him fluids.

Next to the paraquat patient was another man who had swallowed poison: an old, skeletal, toothless man wearing a purple sarong. His legs were tied together to the end of the bed, and his right arm was tied to the side of the bed. He had a drip with atropine (an antidote for many pesticides) going into his other arm, which was tied to the other side of the bed. He was delirious, talking to himself, repeating mindless words, shouting Sinhalese to invisible companions. Jagath explained to me that delirium was the side effect of atropine overdose. The patient had wetted himself, and a pool of urine was on the floor under him. A green blanket was in a bundle partly in the pool of urine. Patients on the other sides, and their relatives, were looking at us to see what was going on, for the paraquat patient was very ill. Nurses in skillfully folded bonnets were going around the ward attending other patients, and there were doctors on the other aisle of the ward.

The desperately ill self-harmers are admitted to what are, for the most part, poorly resourced provincial and local hospitals, where the staff respond to the situation as best they can given the limited resources and expertise available. The patients come in at all times, mostly transferred from peripheral hospitals. In the hospitals where the Paraquat Poisoning Trial was under way, the nurses would typically perform a decontamination routine with each admission, and the patient would be "clerked" by the doctors at the ward, who took a medical history as best they could: What had the patient taken, how much, what are the symptoms of poisoning? The patients' blood pressure and pulse would be recorded, and their eyes checked. Often, if the patient was transferred from another hospital, the information was also taken from the previous medical record.

The process of figuring out what the patient had taken was often an impediment to progress in delivering treatment—the medical records might say one thing, the relatives something else, and patients perhaps were unable to say anything. Without the bottle or receptacle from which the poison came, it was difficult to be sure which poison had been taken, as there are many possibilities. The more unusual products used in self-harm—such as rat poisons, cockroach exterminants, and washing detergents—typically involved a lot of detective work to figure out exactly which compound was producing the presenting pathology. Relatives would be asked to bring the bottle or product into the hospital, and the patient, if remotely conscious, would be quizzed: Where did they get the product? Which brand was it? When did they buy it? Was it bulk-buy strength or diluted and from the *kadee* (small street shop)? Upon arrival, the poisoning patients were seated somewhere to wait for a bed. They were often placed on the veranda unless they were very ill, in which case they were triaged to the inside beds. Patients who had taken organophosphates or paraquat were considered to be in need of more urgent attention. Those who had taken low doses of non-life-threatening drugs were left to recover, and usually they simply sat on a wooden chair somewhere in the busy ward, on a bench on the veranda, or on the floor in the corridor, waiting for the physician to come and send them home the next day.

Adding to the chaos of the admission procedure was the state that the patients were in. They were often still distressed with whatever had prompted them to take poison to begin with, even as they were suffering from the effects of the toxins. Some cried, shouted, or pleaded to be left alone; others stared blankly into the distance or simply slept curled up on the iron beds or on the floor. They certainly received little in the way of comfort, consolation, or counseling. When asked, many doctors and nurses said that poisoning patients needed extra attention due to their psychological-emotional problems, but it was not evident what this meant in practice. Patients rarely questioned the doctors or asked them anything, and the staff rarely explained to them what was being done. Dealing with these patients was often made more difficult by the distressed relatives and friends of the patient, who pleaded with the doctors to do something, begging them to save their relatives' lives.

If the patients were not in an agitated state at the time of arrival at the hospital, they became so after they were made to vomit as part of the decontamination routine.[2] The standard practice in some hospitals was to administer sodium bicarbonate, which would make the patient vomit violently and, most likely, indiscriminately. After the decontamination routine, the doctors and nurses would look after the patients according to the common practice relevant for that particular poison. For many patients, there was not much else for doctors to do other than monitor them for a couple of days. The prognoses were unclear, the toxic effects unknown, and the patients' chances of survival varied depending on the amounts they had ingested as well as what methods of care were available.

The facilities to treat these patients were usually limited. During Salla's fieldwork in the particular hospital where the longest periods of observation were carried out, both drugs and antidotes were often unavailable in the dosages and strengths recommended in the national and international toxicology handbooks—and sometimes they were not available at all. Elsewhere, if the patients were particularly restless they were tied to their beds and thus were unable to clean themselves if they vomited or defecated. Although there seemed to be a lot of staff around on the wards, there were never quite enough of them to keep pace with the needs of a poisoning patient.

In the context of hard-pressed rural health services, self-inflicted injury by rural villagers appeared not to be a high priority. Suicide patients were often treated like the patient described in the vignette earlier. Typically, they might be neglected, scolded, and placed low in the triage that features in the day-to-day running of rural hospitals. A common explanation for this by the doctors in the ward was the lack of facilities. "In places, the patients need ventilators, and we don't have ventilators; that is a real problem we are facing. And ICUs [intensive care units], we have [a] real problem finding ICUs. ICU beds are not available. Yesterday we had one patient admitted with paracetamol overdose, but the antidotes were not available in the ward." In other words, there simply was not a lot that could be done for these patients once they were admitted. Although the explanation for poor treatment was often put down to a lack of facilities and staff, some doctors also alluded to the stigma that suicide patients brought with them:

> Ideally as doctors there shouldn't be any difference between [how we treat] poisoning patients and other patients, but here in Sri Lanka it [poisoning] is a very widespread problem. The medical staff is also a part of the community, they represent the whole community . . . They tend to consider the poisoning patients [with] a little bit less care. I do not mean that they . . . I mean we do all care, but . . . It's difficult to explain. That means that, for example, for every patient we have to treat as humans, we respect them, but regarding this poisoning that respect is little bit lost . . . In the whole community, there are some opinions that they look at poisoning patients as less valuable. I think here we don't intentionally do it, but I think as according to our observation for some part it happens here, it's still here.

Although the doctor is clear about what is expected when it comes to caring for desperately ill poisoning patients, there is also an awareness that the concepts of "value," "respect," and being treated as "human" may be compromised in practice.

Most doctors and nurses argued that poisoning patients had to be treated like everybody else, or even more gently due to their mental trauma. However, in practice these patients often teetered at the very edges of care and compassion. Indeed, some of the practices that patients were subjected to would be unacceptable in other medical regimens, such as the practice of tying patients down or giving them sodium bicarbonate as an emetic. These were the deeply embedded structural and institutional problems that the researchers wished to solve. Through the accumulation of a strong evidence base they hoped to modify the treatment regimens hitherto based on outmoded customs and practices, as well as address public policies in relation to the causes and consequences of attempted suicide.

Research into Poisoning: Where Is the Evidence?

> Dilojan, one of the junior research doctors and a research assistant, took the paraquat patient's pulse and blood pressure. The patient didn't know where he was, he didn't remember being brought over from the primary hospital to the tertiary, but he understood that he was in a hospital. Dilojan had

approached him with the idea of being part of a research study once he had sobered up, at about seven in the morning. Dilojan had told the patient about his condition and the experimental research that might or might not help him. The patient had given his consent. Dilojan checked from Jagath that this was OK to keep him enrolled in the trial even if he didn't know where exactly he was. Jagath said that it was, and he was recruited into the trial. The patient's condition had deteriorated, and by this point it started to be clear that he was going to die. He was no longer talking, he was gasping for air. He had convulsions, shook a lot out of control, and had diarrhea. Shantha, another research assistant, took the patient's blood sugar, and he was given glucose. I asked Jagath what the point was of starting the trial when it was obvious that he was going to die. He said that things had to be done according to the protocol. The patient was put on a drip, and the trial coordinator who was in charge of randomization and blinding brought along the compound that was being tested.

In recent years, toxicology has become a priority area for research in Sri Lanka. The reasons for the past lack of research in this field were associated with an underdeveloped research culture in Sri Lanka in general (Arseculeratne 1999, 2008, 2010), poor communication between local funders and health policy researchers, and a stigma attached to suicide that renders it low on any list of national research priorities. Yet, as many have argued, suicide is a major public health concern that needs to be addressed, and part of this response has been the development of an evidence-based policy in relation to treatment, care, and prevention (Buckley et al. 2004; Eddleston, Sheriff, and Hawton 1998).

The issue caught the attention of international toxicology researchers and clinicians, who started to pay attention to the way that poisoning patients were treated in hospitals in Sri Lanka. "Where is the evidence which tells us why and how these people are dying?" the researchers asked in a provocative article pitched at their peer community of toxicologists (Buckley et al. 2004). To answer these questions, the collaborative network described in chapter 3 brought together international and local researchers with cognate interests to carry out a rigorous enquiry into poisoning. Their aim was to find ways to treat these patients more effectively in the short and long term.

As the subtitle of Buckley et al.'s paper asks, "Is Toxicology Fiddling while the Developing World Burns?" (2004). This was indeed a matter of some urgency. The plight of the poisoning patients as well as the unequal division in health care globally featured as part of a powerful rhetoric driving the formation of the collaboration. Not only did these patients need attention, but the doctors needed to be trained and health care systems given facilities to deal with these admissions. Such research would not only be challenging in practical terms but also ethically fraught.

Given the magnitude of the problem, however, the ethics of not performing the research were an important spur for the researchers involved in the collaboration. As one of the project directors commented, "If it [the research] was easy, everybody would be doing it." The challenge, danger, and discomfort were clearly an attraction, and the work was driven by commitment and a desire to produce positive and beneficent developments with this troubling and tragic problem. The collaboration typified the way in which new configurations of public, private, and charitable funding are being brought together to address health crises and humanitarian biomedicine, often in ways that "transcend certain limitations imposed by the national governance of public health" (Lakoff 2010, 60; also see Biehl 2007; McGoey, Reiss, and Wahlberg 2011).

The trial set up to address paraquat poisoning was carried out in public tertiary care hospital wards. Patients suffering from acute poisoning were recruited into studies on admission to the hospital. When they arrived, clinical research assistants (CRAs) from the "poisoning team" approached the patients. Depending on the patients' condition, they introduced themselves, asked the patients how they were, and began gathering data from them about their condition, but they rarely asked for permission to collect this data. Most patients were included in a cohort study where general data were collected regarding the poisoning and its symptoms. The unusual cases were included in other studies to assess how long the poison would remain in the body; when relevant, the patients were recruited into interventional antidote trials.

The CRAs were not primarily involved in patient management; rather, they were responsible for the collection of clinical data—onto paper records and also on handheld computers from which they regularly uploaded data into the project database. Participant data were collected on different toxicological markers such as blood pressure, pulse, breathing rate, and bowel sounds three times a day for observational studies. Samples of blood and urine were taken for analysis. These data would eventually be tabulated, compared, and inferred from and analyzed locally as well as by researchers outside Sri Lanka. Papers were written for journals with international distribution, and policy proposals were made to international fora on how to improve practice. Based on these findings, local guidelines for treating poisoning patients were improved, and doctors and nurses were encouraged to change their practices.

As such, the work of the researchers has brought into question the standard assumptions about how to deal with these kinds of hospital admissions. A good example in this regard is the use of sodium bicarbonate as an emetic in decontamination of the stomach which is not recommended in international toxicology guidelines (Eddleston and Haggalla 2007; Fernando 2007). As described in chapter 6, many of the poisoning trials began to illuminate further tensions between an evidence-based medicine approach and the prevailing craft-based tradition of clinical practice. As a crucial element in this tension, *abjects* were being recast as *objects* of research.

From Abject to Object to Subject

> The junior doctor research assistants held the paraquat patient while he was having convulsions. The IV drip going to the patient's arm tore his skin; he was bleeding, and some liquid from the drip drizzled out. The patient shook uncontrollably and landed on his side over the edge [of the] bed, drooling, breathing heavily, gasping for air. White, foamy saliva ran down from his mouth to the floor into the growing puddle of IV fluid, urine, and blood. Dilojan, seemingly distressed, said to me that they were having a "helluva time." Friends and relatives stood around looking all this time. Someone was screaming in the background. A guest was vomiting somewhere behind me outside in the garden. I felt utterly useless. I thought that the patient/trial subject was gone, and as morbidly fascinated as I was to see him die, I felt I had to go and sit down. At 10.20 I was told that he had passed away.

Where the patient is in a condition such that treatment is unlikely to be effective, the line between therapy and experiment is a fine one. Carrying out procedures that might bring relief to a dangerously ill patient is one thing; to do so under experimental conditions is quite another. Becoming part of a clinical trial carried out to "global standards" introduces fundamental expectations as to how patients should be treated once they have been designated as research participants or "subjects." Consent, autonomy, and adequate information are cornerstones of international guidelines for human subject research, and they were carefully observed here as well. For admissions that met the trial criteria, consent to participate was a significant hurdle to negotiate. Imparting information about the trial and its design, getting informed consent, securing agreement for the removal of blood samples, and obtaining permission to be contacted for future research—all needed to be accomplished under difficult circumstances.

Out of the eight paraquat poisoning patients who were admitted to the hospital during Salla's participant-observation of the trial, all but one said yes to the invitation to be in the trial. When they were recruited, extra attention was given to the consenting process. Typically, it would take the following form. In the midst of the chaos of an admission, the CRA would try to secure the full attention of the patients by making direct eye contact and addressing them in a serious tone. The aim was to get across unambiguously that what they had ingested was toxic, and that there was an experiment under way that might or might not be able to save them. Taking consent was aimed at the potential participants, but generally it also involved their relatives, who were included in the discussion.

For the actual securing of consent, the researchers had a sheet that they had filled out in advance. It contained boxes to tick and provided information to the effect that the research was to be done by researchers working in a bona fide research collaboration, that refusal would not affect the patient's care, and that they could withdraw from the research at any time even if they had agreed to take part. All the participants needed to do was to sign. On occasion, the participants asked for more information about the research, which was provided to them in an information sheet, or they asked the CRAs what they should do. They were always given a verbal explanation about the experimental nature of the research and told, as on the form, that they could refuse if they wanted and this would not affect their care. Sometimes, the explanations about the side effects of the drugs appeared to be overlooked, as did the fact that randomization might mean they would be in the placebo arm of the trial.

The particular trial we followed was being undertaken because there was some evidence that one particular treatment strategy could have some beneficial effect on outcome in paraquat patients, but this had not yet been verified by means of a randomized clinical trial. The treatments in question were thus not "novel molecular entities" or new products on the market. Although the outcome of the trial was uncertain in terms of outcomes for the participants, being part of a trial did bring a number of benefits. Participants who were enrolled into the trials were subjected to careful monitoring, and many of them received a level of care that was better than they otherwise could have expected as a regular suicide admission to a hospital. They had access to tests and drugs that nonparticipating patients did not. Far from being abjects on the ward, for these patients the heightened protection and attention afforded by the trial and the work of the CRAs increased the likelihood that they would be given "respect, dignity, and be treated like humans," as the doctor put it earlier.

For the participants who found themselves in a trial, the CRAs did not seem different from the other doctors in the wards—they asked more or less the same questions, wrote things down, and examined them. However, the CRAs spent more time with the participants, visited them more frequently, and paid more attention to the details of their self-harm incident and what followed. The research team were told stories about what had preceded the event of taking poison, and sometimes they were approached by the relatives to explain their version of the story and ask about the patient's progress. An empathetic relationship often formed between CRAs, participants, and their families. Being recruited into the trials rendered abjects as objects of scientific experimentation—and, in so doing, they became part of the assemblage of global research governance and were reconfigured as universal human subjects to whom certain standards, protocols, and guidelines apply.

A Precarious Ethics?

The trajectory we have described so far was a linear and largely beneficent one—participant-observation in rural hospitals revealed a series of shifts in the conceptualization of the poisoning patients. Abjects became objects who acquired the status of subjects, who, given their predicament, found themselves in a better position in terms of their care than they would ever have done had the case been otherwise. In the meantime, however, we should not lose sight of the fact that the patients in question were extremely vulnerable.

In 2001, Kenneth Kipnis, on behalf of the U.S. National Bioethics Advisory Commission, created a taxonomy of vulnerability for assessing participants in clinical research. The types of vulnerability he identified were as follows: (1) cognitive, the ability to understand information and make decisions; (2) juridic, being under the legal authority of someone such as a prison warden; (3) deferential, customary obedience to medical or other authority; (4) medical, having an illness for which there is no treatment; (5) allocational, poverty, educational deprivation; and (6) infrastructural limits of the research setting to carry out the protocol. Arguably, the poisoning patients discussed in this article could be considered vulnerable across all these criteria except juridic, because suicide/self-harm is no longer illegal in Sri Lanka. Under these circumstances, the trajectory initiated by clinical research might not always move in the direction of beneficence. Here we enter the realm of precarious ethics.

There is a long and dark history of research on human bodies being carried out in the context of catastrophe or emergency and on populations who are acutely vulnerable. Correctives to these abuses have resulted in numerous protocols and guidelines such as the Declaration of Helsinki (1964), which became the cornerstone of international medical research ethics (World Medical Association 2013). In Sri Lanka, upholding these standards is currently the responsibility of medical faculties and some large hospitals, which now have ethics review committees. Clinical trial protocols are required to undergo such review, and more recently they have had to be registered with a national clinical trials registry.

Yet the situation we are highlighting here is not one in which there is manifest exploitation of the vulnerable by a totalitarian state as in Nazi Germany or by naked commercial interests as in some pharmaceutical trials. On the contrary, there are compelling humanitarian grounds for the intervention. The researchers appear to be driven by the ethos of service and a desire to translate their knowledge into humanitarian benefit rather than any obvious financial gain. They are also aware of the hortatory and often idealistic pronouncements of bioethicists about how to protect the vulnerable in research.

However, as the accounts produced here demonstrate, the gap between idealism and the challenging realities faced by the doctors working in this field is significant (also see Gammelgaard 2004; Yuval and Halon 2000, regarding research on acute myocardial infarction). This is hardly a startling observation, and our purpose in highlighting this gap is not to criticize the extraordinary work that is being performed to produce the evidence that might change policy and practices regarding the treatment of acute poisoning cases. Rather, we would like to open up for scrutiny the points at which the conduct of clinical trials and the wider logic of humanitarian intervention begin to overlap.

As Liisa H. Malkki and others have argued, the logic of humanitarianism can only operate in circumstances where a "bare, naked or minimal humanity" (1996, 390) has been identified (also see Ticktin 2006). Here we are in the realms of extreme poverty, suffering, and misery experienced by those who are physically displaced, politically disenfranchised, and often economically marginalized. For people in such straits, legitimacy, rights, and claims cannot be mobilized through conventional political means; rather, they find their expression in physiological mediations between state, market, population, and, as in the case here, universities and an international community of academic researchers.

For poisoning patients, their involvement in experimental research gives them a visibility that they would not otherwise have had. By drawing attention to the treatment of self-harming poisoning patients in the context of clinical research, we suggest that new ways of managing the relationship between death, rights, and care are brought into view. Taking, or attempting to take, one's own life projects a person into a setting in which they may be treated as an abject, an object, or accorded the respect that goes with the status of a human subject.

Yet we should not overestimate the power or pull of this medical research-cum-humanitarian effort conundrum. The gaze of the clinical trial falls on a relatively small group of self-poisoning admissions, and it stops well short of the broader socioeconomic circumstances of the rural poor whose acts of desperation keep the self-harm statistics at appallingly high rates. As João Biehl (2004) has argued in the context of HIV research in Brazil, some bodies become assimilated into research and the locus of knowledge production and value generation, but the vast majority do not. Similarly, we have highlighted how biomedical experimentation in the context of self-poisoning admissions reveals tensions in the surrounding context: the economics of developing country agriculture, the morality of suicide, and public policy and the humanitarian endeavor. However, biomedical research alone cannot resolve these tensions.

As in other circumstances where medicine is performed in the context of emergency or disaster, concerns arise because of the extreme vulnerability of the research subjects, teetering as they are on the edge of life, society, and its ethics. This aspect of the analysis takes us into a realm of human subject research ethics that we have characterized as precarious. When clinical trials travel globally, particular notions of ethics and research governance travel with them. In this chapter, we have discussed an unusual and perhaps extreme context in which clinical trials are conducted and the ethics of human subject research are invoked. From the Nuremberg Code onward, the laws and guidelines governing human subject research place at their foundation consent, informed and freely given. The normative thrust of these documents is that research participants should not be treated as a corporeal means to scientific ends. On the contrary, they should be seen as persons who must be treated as autonomous subjects with the inviolable right to refuse participation in research.

The trials described here operate at the very edge of such codes. Given the condition at the point of admission to hospital of individuals who have ingested poison, the line between research and therapy is easily blurred, consent taking is at risk of falling short of the ideal, and not all hospital staff share the aspiration to treat the research subject as one to whom a special status should be accorded. Nonetheless, within the normative codes that govern human subject research, there is an expectation that the poisoning patient will move from a state of abjection to one of dignity and respect through the process of becoming a research participant.

Here, falling within an experimental gaze does not result in dehumanization, as it did within the concentration camps. Rather, its opposite occurs: the possibility of recognition as an autonomous and rights-bearing agent. But seeking consent from critically ill patients and their concerned relatives is, as we have shown, a complicated moment. Providing improved regimens of care for these patients is an important moral justification for the trials and one that overrides the potentially fraught moments during which consent is collected. In this moment, incorporating the patients into research and treating them according to international ethics guidelines offered some patients a route back, not only into life itself but into the novel forms of subjectification that arise as part of the global assemblage of biomedical research (see chapter 5). In other contexts of extreme vulnerability, however, we should not underestimate the potential for subjects to become abjects—because ethics is a fragile and precarious business.

Chapter 8

Strategic Ethics

A Regional Collaborative Workshop

Up until this point, our account of collaboration, bioethics, and clinical trials has broadly reflected the views of those who are directly involved in clinical trials. In this penultimate chapter, we situate these accounts within the broader arena of debate that an engagement with international biomedical research brings into play within Sri Lankan society. In these commentaries are expressed yet further readings of clinical trials activity. Rather than collaborative research being seen as an aspect of development, it is singled out as a potential source of a very problematic and persistent underdevelopment. The public debates we document in this chapter were not triggered directly by the trials that we have discussed in previous chapters, but they figure as part of the broader context in which the trials that we studied occurred. In other words, they are a further expression of the work of second-order conceptual and epistemic development needed for trials to become established and accepted. In the cases we document, the idea of just what might be considered to be "ethical" is contested and used strategically and rhetorically to critique and move research cultures in different directions.

To bring these critical voices into play, let us return to the event with which we began this book: the Regional Collaborative Workshop held at the University of Colombo, which posed the question "Why Should We Be Concerned about the Ethics of International Collaboration?" Invitations were widely distributed before the event via a number of regional mailing lists, and the responses were very positive. It appeared that, in many quarters, such an event was seen as both timely and important. The ethics of international science collaborations were clearly of considerable interest.

One person in whose inbox the invitation landed was a philosophy lecturer from Pakistan. Although he could not attend, he e-mailed effusively about the importance of the workshop. Among other things, he spoke of a specific concern: "the irony is that many problems which are actually caused by the process of modernization and ad hoc technological adaptation cannot be resolved without being modernized." What he seemed to be saying was that, for him at least, there was no space outside the terms of the debate as it had already been established; in order to participate, one had to do so in terms of an "other." The location of this workshop and the participation of local representatives talking on the topic of international collaboration appeared to offer the possibility of a small space in which a different dialogue might take place.

Had he attended the workshop, he might have had reasons to be pleased as well as disappointed. He would have been pleased because the event brought together a number of regional perspectives. There were presentations of case studies of international collaboration from Bangladesh, Nepal, India, and Sri Lanka.[1] Open discussion followed about the perils and possibilities inherent in international collaboration. However, he might also have experienced a certain amount of disappointment, for even though the meeting reflected on the ethical issues raised by international collaboration, it did so in terms that mostly kept within an accepted discourse of what these might be and what remedies might be put in place. According to the view he had expressed in his e-mail, he would have encountered the paradox of trying to modernize in order to deal with the problems that modernity itself brings, with the paradox evident in terms of an aspiration to conform to universalistic models of ethical review, research governance, and the notions of the "human subject" that are its focus. There was a good deal of talk about transparency and accountability and a continual return to ethics review by committee as the way to achieve these. The dialogue that took place was instructive, but there was a sense that much was left off the agenda. In the course of the workshop, we began to glimpse some of the tensions evident in the embrace of research as development.

The chair of the Ethics Committee's opening statement at the workshop brought attention to the assumption that biomedical research as a route to development does not automatically mean progress. As suggested by the images he showed concerning the fate of collaborators in France during World War II, collaboration brings cool as well as warm themes. We now explore the potentially adverse consequences of international collaboration by looking at three bioethical controversies that unfolded in Sri Lanka over the period of our fieldwork. These controversies provide a lens through which to view the tensions that occur around the practice of international collaborative research. How people positioned themselves in these disputes revealed the different and often conflicted kinds of investments at work in the business of conducting clinical trials.

It is not our intention to sit in judgment on the controversies we describe. Rather, we would like to consider collaborative research as contributing to "underdevelopment," and the anxieties on which this critique is based.

Postcolonial Critiques

During the workshop, a representative from the Institute for Research and Development in Sri Lanka confronted the chair of the Ethics Committee. The exchange took place after the chair had talked about the ambiguous nature of collaboration. The specific criticism focused on events that followed the 2004 tsunami that swept over several coastal countries in the Asia-Pacific region on Boxing Day. At the time, a flurry of humanitarian aid organizations had introduced research and rehabilitation programs in Sri Lanka without sufficient standards for doing research under such circumstances. As noted by several anthropologists who have studied disasters and humanitarian aid (e.g., Fassin 2012; Pfeiffer 2003; E. Simpson 2014; Ticktin 2006), when a crisis sets in motion activity that is ostensibly about relief and assistance, it simultaneously generates a reality of its own—during the commotion, other things can happen. In 2004 a Japanese collaboration had conducted research in Sri Lanka and had taken samples from people in order to study post-traumatic stress disorder.

In this instance, the allegation was that the study of post-traumatic stress disorder was both opportunistic and extractive: the traumatized individuals who had been displaced by the flood provided blood samples to foreign researchers without any clear indication of why or to what end. In the wake of the disaster, these people were far too vulnerable to be included in research, yet the samples were collected and shipped out of the country. Their removal raised further concerns about illegal appropriation of samples and "biopiracy." Finally, came the most serious allegation: the collection of samples from vulnerable people would not have happened were it not for the questionable ethics clearance that had been given. The approval, it was alleged, was invalid as it was given post hoc; moreover, it was nepotistic as there was a family connection between one of the researchers and a member of ethics committee. These views expressed from the floor were part of the wider critique of international research collaborations (e.g., Sumathipala 2006), which have pointed to some as the development equivalent of iatrogenic medicine.

The audience, mostly composed of researchers from prestigious medical faculties across the island, quickly silenced the questioner, and made it clear that they were unhappy and uncomfortable with the public airing of these allegations. For them, the tsunami and the chaos it wrought—not only to people and places, but also to their procedures and protections—were problems of the past, and they considered the case closed. Some expressed the view that the study in question did indeed have legitimate ethics clearance from an appropriately constituted local ethics committee, so they did not see why the issue needed to be revisited again.

There was a general feeling that the grievances went much deeper than samples and consent in that particular study, connecting with a much wider and more critical analysis of the role of international biomedical collaborations in Sri Lanka. And, in the context of the workshop, many saw such views as unhelpful for progressing discussions about how to conduct ethics reviews and, by extension, legitimate scientific research.

The Institute for Research and Development (IRD), which the speaker from the floor represented, is an independent research organization.[2] The events surrounding the tsunami had led members of the IRD to produce a corpus of materials regarding mental health research (Allden et al. 2009; Ekanayake et al. 2013), disaster management (Siriwardhana et al.

2012; Sumathipala, Jafarey, et al. 2010), and bioethics (Sumathipala 2006; Sumathipala, Siribaddana, et al. 2010). They drafted guidelines for research activity that takes place during or after a disaster (Sumathipala, Jafarey, et al. 2010; Sumathipala, Siribaddana, and Patel 2004). For their bioethics work, the group was funded by the Wellcome Trust, and they published several articles on the skills and views of ethics committee members (Sumathipala et al. 2008) as well as research participants' understandings of informed consent and their role as research subjects (Sumathipala, Siribaddana, et al. 2010). In contexts where scientific literacy is low and trust in doctors is high among the research participants, Sumathipala and Siribaddana also suggested the value of a research ombudsman, whose role it would be to ascertain whether consent was freely given, autonomous, and without therapeutic misconception in contested cases (Sumathipala and Siribaddana 2004; also see Simpson 2005). This move would, in effect, introduce people to watch over the people watching over.

The notions of research governance that IRD members put forward mirror the organization's advocacy for social justice and progressive change in Sri Lanka. Their particular interest is in the role of science, research, and development in reaching these objectives. As their website at the time of our research stated, one of their aims is "to create a new strategic alliance among academics, scholars, professionals, and the public to build a new research culture in Sri Lanka, so that the power of knowledge in science & technology could be mobilized to address the problems of the society using an evidence-based approach, which in turn is crucial for the sustainable development of the country" (Institute for Research and Development 2014). Not surprisingly, international collaboration in the form of "strategic partnerships" is an area of great interest and concern for the IRD. Research is seen as welcome when it can be harnessed to the needs of the society and its people; research according to this definition ought to produce development in the classic sense. The organization is critical when they see research as extractive, harmful, and serving the interests of Western—or indeed local—elites.

Their stance is not antiscience or anti-Western per se but rather a continual questioning of whether knowledge has application and value locally. The word "locally" here references far more than the local science community—it extends to the user-beneficiaries of the knowledge produced. Their disaster management guidelines make this view explicit: "More stringent policies have to be followed to prevent unethical data collection and exploitation of

disaster survivors giving due attention to issues such as a) what types of research, b) how soon, c) if based on local needs and priorities and d) complexities when combined with aid and clinical care" (Sumathipala, Jafarey,
et al. 2010, 128). In this view, research carried out under circumstances of
emergency is not denied outright, but it should only be done within stringent frameworks and with careful consideration of the needs of those whose
very predicament is what renders them of scientific interest.

Research, when conducted for needs that are scientific rather than applied,
and distant rather than local, is brought into question because it might be
exploitative and potentially harmful. This is reflected in the IRD's disaster
guidelines:

> In the long-term disaster period, the IRD experienced the influx of foreign
> academics and researchers intent on conducting various researches on these
> Tsunami-affected populations and saw how beneficial and detrimental
> these can be on the local populations. Many of the researchers were from the
> developed world and their research agendas and interventions based on
> the western perspective which acted negatively on the local vulnerable popu-
> lations. (Sumathipala, Jafarey, et al. 2010, 125)

From this perspective, local researchers are seen as those best able to gauge
the needs of local people and how those needs might be best served by research. International collaborations and researchers are seen to promote foreign interests and cause local harms. The work of foreigners, even when they
work with local researchers, may not bring benefits to "local people." This
argument is one that promotes a particular vision of research culture in which
research is not in itself problematic unless it is a neocolonial, top-down exercise that furthers foreign research interests.

When international collaborative clinical trials are conducted in resource-
poor contexts in different parts of the world, public controversies have followed, and fundamental discontents have increasingly found expression in
the language of bioethics. In the Sri Lankan case, the possibility of research
as underdevelopment was captured in the critique of Western biomedical research collaborations and the institutional grounds from which they spring.
Such critiques are pronationalist and left-leaning in their orientation, and
they echo postcolonial and Marxist analyses of the role of external powers
and forces in regional development. Targeting the commercial aspects of the

clinical trials gives bioethics a strongly political hue, representing a novel front on which an old battle can be fought.

The Disbanding of an Ethics Committee

The second controversy demonstrated how disputes surrounding medical research are not limited to displeasure with foreigners working in international collaborations within Sri Lanka but also feature in the local institutional landscape. As reported on March 4, 2012, in the *Sunday Leader,* an English-language newspaper in Sri Lanka, the ethics committee of a university medical faculty was disbanded by its dean of medicine (Wickrematunge 2012).

As described in the article, several protocols pertaining to a pharmaceutical company's multisite randomized controlled trial (RCT) were submitted to the university's ethics review committee, but their approval was delayed. According to the article, in the meeting where the submissions were discussed, some of the applications were accepted but some were deemed to need expert opinion for further assessment. The committee then adjourned to give the reviewers sufficient time to complete their work. What made the item newsworthy was that the committee needed more time for the review than was available before the next meeting. Also, although it was not explicitly stated in the news article, clinical trial protocol submissions have deadlines; if they are not granted ethics clearance within certain time frames, they run the risk of being lost to competing groups in the country or elsewhere. The delay potentially put the committee in a bad light as it threatened to jeopardize the interests of the pharmaceutical company that wished to perform the trials.

Soon after the meeting, the Dean of the Medical Faculty announced that the ethics committee was incompetent in its decision making. The dean and a number of other members of the faculty were displeased with the way that the ethics committee was reviewing applications for ethics clearance. The changes requested by the committee, they said, reflected a lack of understanding of the multisite nature of pharmaceutical company trials, whereby methodologies and outcomes should remain in conformity with globally established standards and not be changed by individual local ethics committees—the trials had, after all, already been approved by ethics committees in other countries. By requesting changes to these protocols the local ethics committee was seen as overreaching its remit and engaging with the science of the RCTs rather than focusing on the ethics of subject protection per se. After an acrimonious wrangle, the ethics committee was dismissed, a new committee was put in place, and eventually the trials were approved.

The chair of the disbanded ethics committee believed the dean had overstepped his authority by disbanding their committee, so she went public with the dean's actions. A crucial element in her case was that the dean had close associations with a research unit that was hoping to host the trials. This was, in her view, a fundamental conflict of interest—as an important part of the research assemblage, the dean should have removed himself from handling matters relating to the trials altogether.

Our intention is not to take sides in this dispute—indeed, we have sketched only a very general picture of what was a complex, multilayered conflict—but to identify key vectors and conceptual issues that emerged. The episode illuminated starkly different visions of what the prevailing research culture should be and how it should be governed. In an interview, a member of the disbanded ethics committee explained her concerns regarding the use of placebos in one of the pharmaceutical company trials, an area where the ethics committee and the sponsors disagreed in what they felt was appropriate use. The committee also had concerns about the participant information sheets for the trial, which were lengthy and written in language that they thought people would not be able to understand:

> Our people [i.e., Sri Lankans] are not going to read the whole thing and ask questions, they will just sign for whatever that is written in the information sheet and give consent, so it was really unfair when they were subjected to this kind of sort of thing. They were abusing their ignorance as well as their compliance to whatever the doctors suggest because actually they see them as gods. We are abusing such situations.

For this former ethics committee member, the primary duty of the committee is to consider the safety of the Sri Lankan population. This did not mean a wholesale condemnation of research, however:

> I am not against clinical trials, without clinical trials we do not have the advancement in pharmacology, but these are funded by commercial industries, so there are ethical issues in relation to those. There are other trials which are conducted purely in the genuine interest, and such trials we need to

promote. I don't know the ethics of these because these are industry-funded. Maybe if the mentioned issues were cleared and by obtaining a second opinion, and if the second opinion also was in favor of granting clearance, we would have done it—we have no objections. Some people probably think that we are against clinical trials, but that is not the case. I think we should conduct clinical trials, but not with the intension of making money but with a benefit for the country as well as maybe the population largely.

The quote highlights the critical differences between clinical trials sponsored by commercial enterprises and publicly funded, investigator-led trials. There is a suspicion that the former do not prioritize the interests of the trial participants and that they are conducted solely with monetary interests in mind rather than a benefit to Sri Lankans. A recurring theme in the Sri Lankan arguments against pharmaceutical companies conducting trials in resource-poor countries has been the precarious financial situation of the study participants and the consequent potential for exploitation. In highlighting the ethical problems with this particular set of pharmaceutical company trials, the committee's stance was presented to us as an honorable and ethical one. That they were disbanded as a result was felt to be a misuse of power that put the safety of the people of Sri Lanka at risk.

The *Sunday Leader* article also cited the dean's view of the furor, saying that the trials funded by pharmaceutical companies had nothing to do with the decision to disband the ethics committee; rather, the faculty had lost confidence in the committee because of its persistent delays, internal conflicts, and resignations. He said that he had a petition signed by fifty people on the faculty who supported his decision.

In another interview, a senior researcher from the Faculty at the heart of the dispute—said that they did want to attract more research to Sri Lanka: "We have the potential because we have such good science to provide careers and make internationally valid science. We have had troubles like war and the global recession, but we can still try and push for visibility at scientific meetings and improve our track record. We have only begun to scratch the surface." The dean was also publicly advocating for what he believed to be crucial to the realization of this potential: a smoothly functioning regulatory system that facilitated all research, including studies carried out by pharmaceutical companies. The scope of this opportunity was not only institutional but national.

A group of individuals, including members of the faculty, drafted a national law on clinical trials in 2011. The *Sunday Leader* article spoke with another senior member of the unit who emphasized the global reach of local research and the role of the new legislation in it: "The aim of the new Sri Lankan Clinical Drug Act is to regulate the industry and bring it in line with international standards." In short, to be successful, the multisite trials needed to proceed in step with global standards; in order to gain universally acceptable data, the protocols needed to be observed and not changed in the process. As we argued in chapter 7, to put Sri Lanka on the international biomedical research map, it is necessary to create confidence that research carried out there is the same as it is anywhere else in the world. Harmonized, working regulatory standards are a crucial part of a functioning trial environment that can take its place in a multisite, global, RCT laboratory. In this view, expressions of local specificity can easily prove an impediment to efforts to achieve this objective (Simpson et al. 2015).

The example of the disbanded ethics committee points to the varying concepts of what a national knowledge economy should look like and what the role of ethics review should be within it. What kind of research should be supported? Who should fund it? How and by whom should it be overseen and regulated? The attempt to draft a national law on clinical trial regulation also raised these questions, and as of the time of this writing it was still proving to be a complicated and protracted process (Karunanayake 2012; Lang and Siribaddana 2012).

The proposed regulatory act identified the Ministry of Finance as the key authority overseeing clinical trials instead of the Ministry of Health. This move—ostensibly a move from a health interest to a financial interest—was controversial in the eyes of many. Critics objected to the proposed legislation on the grounds that they had never seen a draft of the act so the majority of the scientific community could not stand behind it. The Sri Lankan Clinical Trials Sub-Committee of the National Medicines Regulatory Authority were so displeased about the Ministry of Finance becoming the authorizing body that they resigned over the disagreement. As they saw it, they could not approve of this linkage to a financially driven research culture. The proposals regarding which ministry should oversee clinical trials were subsequently withdrawn, and the Ministry of Health was reinstated. In 2012, the law was proposed to parliament, but its progress has stalled. As of 2017, there had been no further progress.

A Dispute over Findings

Controversies in science are rarely simple disputes about facts; often they represent deeper contests over meaning, interpretation, and how these should be applied in practice (Collins 2014; Mazur 1975, 1981; Nelkin 1984; Nowotny and Hirsch 1980; Suryanarayanan and Kleinman 2013). In our third example, we consider another instance in which an international collaboration sparked public debate, resulting in a local reconfiguration of biomedical research and its ethics. The controversy initially grew out of a series of publications in *The Lancet* that each analyzed the same condition but reported very different results.

In the making of scientific claims, a number of registers are brought into play. The journal articles in question reported on research into different ways of treating poisoning by oleander and organophosphates (a group of pesticides). Given the presumed scientific rigor of RCTs, a variety of questions are raised when different results are produced in relation to what is ostensibly the same phenomenon. Typically, these questions focus on experimental inaccuracies, differences in populations, and inadequacies in the way that the tools and technologies of the researcher's trade have been used. However, by drawing attention to the socio-cultural contexts in which knowledge is made, we suggest that there might be something more going on here than research lacking in rigor. What this dispute highlighted is the way that local critiques of clinical trials activity become inflected with interests that are at once personal and ethical as well as political and scientific.

In the 1990s and 2000s, two significant research groups were working on poisoning in Sri Lanka. Each studied a range of poisons and how they are best dealt with. The researchers were, at times, working on the same conditions and substances.

Oleander is a bushy tree that grows widely across Sri Lanka, and its flowers and fruit affect the heart's functioning when ingested; oleander poisoning is lethal in up to 10 percent of cases (Eddleston et al. 1999). Pacemakers had been the accepted way to address the cardiac arrhythmias that follow acute oleander poisoning, but these devices were not always available in the rural hospitals where these poisoning patients were likely to present (Eddleston et al. 2000). In 2000, a British doctor working in Sri Lanka and his group published an article that suggested that an antidote to oleander poisoning called antidigoxin fab could be an effective alternative to the use of pacemakers.

In 2003, another group published an article suggesting that activated charcoal was a cheaper and more efficient way of treating the heart problems caused by the ingestion of oleander (de Silva et al. 2003). Charcoal activated with oxygen to increase its surface area was believed to absorb the ingested poison effectively, enabling it to pass through the digestive system without being absorbed and thereby reducing its clinical effects.

Meanwhile, the first group had a study in progress that suggested that treatment with activated charcoal was ineffective in preventing death due to organophosphates (pesticides) and yellow oleander (Eddleston et al. 2008). The study, which was funded by the Wellcome Trust, was one of a number of high-profile collaborations between Oxford University in the United Kingdom and the University of Colombo in Sri Lanka. Both universities had provided this study with ethics clearance. In 2003, while the trial was still in progress, its ethics were called into question, and controversy ensued.

We interviewed the study's principal investigator, and he described the background of the controversy:

> One day we found a statement in the medical notes of a patient that a clinician had come to see a patient whose bowels were not looking very good and the question was if the charcoal had caused an acute surgical abdomen. So he came to see the patient and wrote to the notes something along the lines of: "This patient is being poisoned by charcoal in an unethical clinical trial, and I'm not willing to take any responsibility because this patient is unethically trialed. I'll be writing to the medical secretary in Colombo, to express my displeasure" . . . I was advised by Sri Lankan colleagues to sit it out. Unfortunately, soon after, I was out of town in Colombo when it happened, I was called by one of my research staff at seven o'clock in the morning about a newspaper story about the study.

It transpired that the incident with the patient had been reported in two local newspapers with the claim that the trial was killing patients with a "black chemical."[3] The principal investigator continued:

> I think the patient died about Saturday morning. By then, he had been in the hospital for 12 hours. Afterwards, the surgeon had gone to see the body with a judicial medical officer, the coroner, and a reporter, and they made the decision that I killed the patient and it should go to the newspapers . . . It

was published in the newspapers and the radio the next day. The coroner wrote to the hospital to say that you must stop this trial. Now, the coroner's role, in my understanding, is to investigate what happened. If he feels that a police case has happened, he would appeal that case to the magistrate. Then the court of law will investigate the case and make the decision to arrest the doctor or whatever. But instead he wrote to the hospital and said that you must stop this trial, this trial is unethical. Killing patients.

Following the newspaper reports, demonstrations against the trial were held near the hospital where the study was conducted.[4] Reported in the newspaper articles were the concerns of the participants' relatives, who claimed that they had signed the consent form thinking they were consenting to treatment rather than research and that the patient had died because of the activated charcoal he had received rather than the ingested poison.

The principal investigator also explained that an issue further animating the controversy was the use of gastric lavage for poisoning patients. He explained that this was not the standard recommendation in international toxicology guidelines, but it was nonetheless widely practiced in Sri Lanka. His assessment was that lavage was common because it was seen to be "doing something," even though in many cases it proved to do more harm than good. For this reason, the principal investigator had opted not to perform lavage on the trial participants, which gave the families an impression of neglect—even though this was widely recognized as part of the "best available treatment" in such cases.

After the furor over the death of the patient, several other sites where the study was conducted were still willing to continue the research. However, despite the attempts to reassure the public by explaining the therapeutic role of charcoal in organophosphate poisonings, the principal investigator said the credibility of the research had been badly damaged:

> The doctor who instigated the event went to the Government Medical Officers' Association [G.M.O.A] with a delegate to vouch the study to be halted. I got an overnight bus to Colombo, and by 8 a.m. I was sitting outside the secretary of health's office. When he arrived, he said, "The G.M.O.A. sent a delegation to my office yesterday" and they said, "If you don't stop this trial now we'll strike nationally." And he said, "What can I say when they put something like that to me; you can't compete."

Faced with the possibility of the entire country's clinical staff going on strike, the researcher stopped the trial.

By the time Salla was working in Sri Lanka, the heat of the controversy had cooled. Nonetheless, the events had significant consequences for how trial sites were organized and particularly where new international collaborations were formed. Among the senior researchers it was said that "no white face should enter the trial site [where the controversy had taken place]." Although these comments were often made in jest, they were part of a more considered policy decision on the part of the research group managers. It was felt that sending in foreign investigators for short visits could cause confusion over the leadership of the trial. It was also felt that this strategy would help effect a meaningful transition to local leadership of the trials. In line with this position, also Salla's requests to visit the hospital were politely put aside. The publicity surrounding the death of the trial participant had clearly left deep and abiding suspicions about international researchers in the institutional memory of the hospital where the trials had taken place.

We attempted to look beyond the public furor by discussing it with some of the protagonists. Significantly, a key issue identified in the various attempts to explain the course of events was the social relations existing within and between the international research collaborations. Nobody thought that the ethical concerns raised about the trial in the press were the primary reason for the controversy. A view put forward by several doctors and researchers was that research ethics were not really behind the media frenzy, but rather the conflicts over scientific relationships between the groups in which the research was being conducted.

A Sri Lankan researcher, who had worked in the hospital at the time when the events unfolded, reflected on the controversy as follows:

> I think it was about the seniors of the researchers. The seniors in two British universities didn't get along. Collaboration happens basically because Sri Lankans travel abroad and make friendships; they have contacts which they bring back because of personal interests . . . I was a house officer [a junior doctor] at the time in the hospital where these studies were made and sort of in between the two teams. I got along with both sides but was told by the head of my research team, "You can co-operate with them, but you have to follow me," basically. There had been tensions in research between these two groups, and they were competing.

The researcher suggested that the controversy around the death of the patient went beyond the individuals involved and into the wider politics of international collaboration. Competition, rather than collaboration, seemed to
be the primary driver for relationships:

> *Sri Lankan researcher (SLR)*: People feel like they can't trust each
> other—their feelings and ideas would be stolen, other people
> publish them first. Both the teams were working on similar
> things. Then when the results were published, one study was in
> favor and one was against.
>
> *Salla Sariola (SS)*: How do you explain that?
>
> *SLR*: Well, I can't, we can't know which one is correct. I suppose we
> need a new study to see about that.
>
> *SS*: So science is getting in the way of human relationships.
>
> *SLR*: Yes, or human relationships are getting on the way of science!

Several researchers made similar comments to the effect that competitive relationships were an impediment to collaborative knowledge production. As
Bruno Latour (1982, 1993) would have it, research is not a "pure" emergence
of facts but is deeply entangled in the circumstances that led to their investigation in the first place. In this process, the relationships between the people
working on the research are not without relevance; rather, they play an important part in understanding the way in which the results of biomedical science are shaped and situated. As Brian Martin (2005) has argued, scientific
evidence on its own can never resolve a scientific controversy—only people
can. Martin has maintained that "evidence can always be disputed and theories are always open to revision, so disputes can persist so long as participants are willing to pursue them" (Martin 2005, 38).

In this case, new large grants and changes in leadership led to different
organizational approaches to research and collaboration. A professor of clinical toxicology, who was appointed as the director, explained how to get
collaboration right in this context where relations were fraught and can "get
in the way of science":

> So you know, if you start to look at clinical research you do have to work out
> who are the active, existing participants [in the field of research], who's going
> to drive the bus, and who are the passengers. It's very important for them to

get on the bus and understand where it's going, even when you may not expect very much out of them. And then those who are observers, and there are a lot of observers, they're important as well. The observers are more like observers who happen to be observing you from the front of the bus, who you might end up figuratively driving over [if you're not careful]. It's worthwhile maintaining good collaborations rather than going to new hospitals with a lot of patients and having to establish new relationships there, because you have to deal with the complexity of people's interpersonal relationships which can flip-flop around in this country.

The director further suggested that to get research "right," careful attention has to be given to social relations in the location of the research. He suggested that for successful collaboration at country level, one needs to know the power dynamics of the local research "field." Not doing so is to generate the potential for mistrust, fear, confusion, and competition. It might also encourage power games and ethical malpractice; in extreme situations, it may put researchers at risk of harm.

Yet carefully managed collaborations can result in warmer themes. Several years down the line from the controversy over the aborted poisoning trial, new channels for dialogue had opened up between the two groups. The reframing of mutual interests led them to decide that it was better to merge their research interests, not the least because they were often bidding for the same sources of funding. In effect, with the changing of personnel, the conflict was dissolved rather than resolved.

Scandals and deep divisions are as common in the world of Sri Lankan biomedical research as they are anywhere. For researchers coming from outside the country and its networks, it takes time to work out the existing relationships. The aborted trial example shows just how volatile these relationships can be and how they can undermine research and lead to contested findings. Indeed, it appears that "ethics" plays a strategic role in such disputes—it is a means to other ends. Conducting ethical research in transnational settings is a complex business, and if shortcomings are identified, these can be used by others to water down the value and credibility of otherwise legitimate scientific practice. They can also be used as a means of distraction. The cry of "ethics malpractice," it turns out, may have little to do with the protection of the participants, and more to do with the mutual positioning of different collaborative ventures both locally and internationally.

Bioethics and Controversy

The history of bioethics is one of controversies. As scientific research in medicine becomes more globalized and its methods travel, "it is to be expected that its controversies will also be globalised" (Martin 2008). The events we have described in this chapter make explicit how a growing engagement with biomedical research generates different visions of how this activity fits into the wider imaginaries of culture, economy, and nation. As analytic devices, these controversies throw light on what is at stake for different protagonists. Disputes over just what a national research culture should look like bring the different positions into the fore.

Controversies make people reflect upon and rethink their positions, aspirations, and motivations with regards to collaboration, clinical trials, and bioethics. In scientometric measurements, research cultures are often spoken of as though they are fully harmonized national knowledge systems (e.g., Wagner 2008). However, what should be clear by now is that this simply is not the case—development through engagement with international biomedical science collaborations is complex and splintered. There is no single, common objective for international research collaboration. In Anna Tsing's words, "in transnational collaborations overlapping but discrepant forms of cosmopolitanism may inform contributions allowing them to converse, but across difference" (Tsing 2004, 13). In the examples we have discussed in this chapter, conflicts arose from the fact that people had discrepant ideas about the relationship between good scientific conduct and the ethics by which it should be governed and guided. All this goes beyond any simple right or wrong way to conduct collaborative research.

Differences in views about research and its regulation render the machinery of ethical governance differently visible both to the public and the disputants (Martin and Richards 1995). After we had carried out fieldwork in Sri Lanka over a number of years, it became apparent that the world of international biomedical science collaborations is highly factionalized, with loyalties often based on intellectual pedigrees and underscored by networks in which kinship, ethnicity, and religion play important roles. When striking up international collaborative relationships, overseas partners are often unaware of the complexity of the local landscape. When controversies erupt, matters of disagreement surpass individual opinions, and conflicts are used to channel other registers of difference. In the controversies that we have described here, the stakes were often so high that attempts at tempered public debate had little impact.

Thus, contrary to the presumption that there is a lack of research governance in low-income countries, Sri Lanka demonstrates something of an excess of competing authorities, formulations, and ideas of how regulation works and in whose interests. In short, there are different moral and political authorities in play when it comes to the legitimation of ethical review and oversight. The principles on which they rely draw their authority from different regulatory regimes and ethical traditions, and they manifest in procedures that are far from harmonized in practice. This poses the all-important question: which voices prevail?

The close connection between controversies in biomedical research, ethics, and power allows certain positions to become dominant over others. Those who have organizational and cultural capital are able to set up regulatory structures that are conducive to their interests. In the absence of either a uniform governance structure or a law governing the conduct of clinical trials, there is scope for individuals or groups to fill that space with initiatives that may look very similar to one another on the surface but are very different in practice. This fluidity can be a source of "underdevelopment," with governance being compartmentalized and remaining incoherent.

In the fractured governance landscapes we encountered, invocation of the ethical was often used as a means to criticize others. (As a human rights lawyer we interviewed once put it to us, "the law has failed, the constitution has failed, let's give bioethics a try.") Under the novel guise of concerns over bioethics, interests of a political and, indeed, a personal nature could be aired. Although expressed in the language of subject protection, promotion of justice, and the mitigation of inequality, relations on the ground were characterized by allegations of neocolonialism, unfair competition, and plagiarism. In more serious cases, such allegations gave way to accusations of nepotism, corruption, "biopiracy," and scientific fraud. In this power play, what ethics "is" matters less than what it can "do."

In the allegations of unethical research conduct that we have reported on here, a common theme is that one set of researchers stood to benefit in some way from making others look as though they had acted unethically or improperly. Science and bioethics collaborations are not simply about cooperation but also provide platforms on which to fight other battles, gain scientific merit, and further careers. They are also important mechanisms for the development of normative structures and the emergence of new conceptual frameworks. The examples we have provided show that conventional accounts of the place of research in "development" and as "progress" fail to recognize the importance of these local conflicts and negotiations in rendering new ideas and practices into the vernacular.

Chapter 9

RESEARCH AS DEVELOPMENT

Unintended Consequences

In this book, we set out to describe ethnographically the entanglement of biomedical research with a variety of development objectives in contemporary Sri Lanka. This entanglement has been seen to unfold at a variety of relational scales, ranging from the personal through the institutional and into national and international arenas. The practices through which we explored the dynamics of biomedical research and development were those of clinical trials, collaboration, and bioethics. Methodological engagement with these practices has drawn attention to the manner of their assimilation into the Sri Lankan setting. By way of conclusion, we offer some further reflections on the relationships between these practices and the implications that this study has for biomedical research as development in other parts of the global south.

Bioethics and Clinical Trials

Bioethics is a distinctive and important thread woven into the global reach of biomedical experimentation involving humans, and it is no less so in the account we have given here. The lexicon of bioethics has been built around foundational concepts such as autonomy, dignity, respect, voluntarism, beneficence, and justice (Anderson and Steneck 2011; De Vries, Rott, and Paruchuri 2011), and these terms feature in the cogitations surrounding engagement with clinical trials in Sri Lanka that we have developed here. As Renée Fox argued long ago, this lexicon gives bioethics a distinct orientation and accords "paramount status to the value complex of individualism, underscoring the principles of individual rights, autonomy, self-determination, and their legal expression in the jurisprudential notion of privacy" (1990, 206). The development of this perspective reached a kind of florescence in the approach referred to as "principlism." Using the four cardinal points of justice, beneficence, non-maleficence, and autonomy, it was believed that bioethicists could navigate their way through the kinds of problems that progress in biomedicine were increasingly throwing up (Beauchamp and Childress 1989). This formulation—"the Georgetown mantra," as it became known—has been used widely. Indeed, one of the reasons we refer to it here, thirty years after it was brought into existence, is that it was still in use for teaching medical ethics in Sri Lanka at the time of our fieldwork.

In the clinical trials assemblage, the conceptual architecture that has been drawn on has as its central tenets informed consent (what it is, how it might be meaningfully elicited, and how it might best be rendered "informed"); subject protection (how the aspirations of trialists might be balanced against the acceptable risks to participants); and questions of benefit (how much, to whom, and to what ends). In taking on the responsibility of performing a trial, conformity to the latest standards and directives is crucial. Moreover, these standards and directives are shaped by the deliberations of those who make up the ranks of bioethicists—philosophers, lawyers, doctors, and social scientists working in collaboration with government and industry regulators. As most of these individuals tend to be drawn from countries in the global north, the conceptual underpinnings of bioethics are mostly consistent with those in play in those parts of the world. Clinical trial regulatory tools, such as the International Conference on Harmonization Good Clinical Practice Guidelines (ICH-GCP), thus operate with considerable hege-monic force. This force is most readily apparent across sites in the global south where the conceptual and material infrastructures are least developed.

The guidelines lay out "a more economical use of human, animal and ma-terial resources, and the elimination of unnecessary delay in the global de-velopment and availability of new medicines whilst maintaining safeguards on quality, safety and efficacy, and regulatory obligations to protect public health" (Dixon 1998). Yet bringing together a genealogy of universal human rights with commercial pharmaceutical research interests has raised suspi-cions about the role of ethical oversight in research (Abraham 2007; Abra-ham and Reed 2002). Is the work of oversight the handmaiden rather than the governor of trial activity? And does it perform a role that is essentially procedural, bureaucratic, and rule observing (Stark 2011)? Is there a space in which bioethics might operate that is not already hedged about with these parameters?

As the field of expertise that sets out to understand the relationship be-tween Western biomedical knowledge and human value systems, bioethics covers a very wide terrain. However, given its particular genealogy, it is hardly surprising that bioethics brings about particular problems when it travels be-yond the human value system out of which it emerged. As we have demon-strated, the standardized, technical specifications underpinning the safe and ethical conduct of a trial are one thing, but just how these articulate with the domain of ethics as constituted in the local setting is quite another. Echo-ing Arthur Kleinman, we see people's moral realities as being shaped by local experience whereas bioethics is "translocal"—that is, it is "a view from nowhere" rather than a view from somewhere (Kleinman 1995, 2006; also see Muller 1994). As Jessica Muller once put it, "rationalistic thinking and a deductive utilitarian orientation to problem solving provide an illusion of ob-jectivity and logic. Informed by the legacy of Cartesian duality, the analyti-cal style of bioethics contributes to a distancing of moral discourse from the complicated settings and interactions within which moral dilemmas are cul-turally constructed, negotiated and lived" (1994, 52). In contexts of poverty and underdevelopment, this point is of even greater consequence as it sits within the broader issues of injustice and abuses of power. Indeed, the con-ceptual infrastructure of bioethics that underpins the governance and regu-lation of clinical trials can operate as a device to convert collective local concerns into ones that are individualized, procedural, and uncontentious. As we argue in the final section of this chapter, bioethics appears to be operating rather like Ferguson's notion of an anti-politics machine, in that it serves to draw parameters around what is and is not of actionable concern when operating in a low-income setting (Ferguson 1994). Before exploring this point further, however, we must square a particular circle.

The quest for standardization, consistency, and universality in the use and meaning of terms and concepts is integral to the quest for a global bioethics. Yet the aspiration for a singularity of sorts must always confront a plurality of local visions. Attempts to square this particular circle have resulted in some acrimonious but nonetheless healthy debate around the status of local voices and sensitivities in the global bioethics assemblage (Bracanovic 2013, in response to Chattopadhyay and De Vries 2008; Chattopadhyay and De Vries 2013; Ten Have and Gordijn 2011). One obvious conclusion to be drawn from these debates is that at the point of confluence between the global and local, there is work to be done regarding the management of "engaged universals" (Tsing 2004). Our contention here is that there ought to be better opportunities for voices from the global south to shape the terms of north–south engagements where biomedical research is concerned.

In our account, we have tried to provide examples of how researchers in Sri Lanka became part of the global bioethics and clinical trials assemblages and did so by appropriating and reappropriating its ideas and practices in the day-to-day work of installing ethics committees, providing ethics training, building clinical trials capacity, and introducing novel transactions such as informed consent procedures to be used in trials. These appropriations show that there is indeed a relationship between Kleinman's "nowhere" and our "somewhere," and furthermore that the distinction may, in any case, be of limited utility. The somewhere of an international clinical trial is, we would argue, increasingly evident in the "nowhere" of bioethics, as the plain facts of cultural diversity, ethnic pluralism, and structural inequality begin to reshape an apparently fixed and hegemonic conceptual architecture—or what we referred to in chapter 6 as science in mode 2^n. To appreciate the importance of this point fully, we need to look more closely at the fabric of social and cultural interactions that make up the day-to-day running of a trial—the sociality of experimentation.

Clinical Trials and Collaboration

The chemist and philosopher Michael Polanyi went to great lengths in his explication of "personal knowledge" to argue that the making and valida- tion of knowledge cannot be understood as wholly distinct from the emo- tional and spiritual interiors of those whose task it is to create and validate such knowledge (Polanyi 1958). In turn, these interiors are shaped by the re- lationships that make up the social worlds in and out of which scientific practice evolves. Rather like Latour's critique of the pure emergence of facts (1982, 1993), Polanyi's treatise was a wide-ranging critique of what he saw as a "naïve objectivism" that underpins the view that the only valid scientific knowledge is that which emerges out of methods that are demonstrably im- personal, explicit, and easily captured in textual representation. What Po- lanyi was seeking to highlight was not only the importance of the tacit and inarticulate dimensions of how we come to know but also the role of relation- ships, mutuality, and trust in scientific pursuit. All this he gathered together under the heading of "conviviality," drawing attention to the continued em- beddedness of these vectors in scientific practice and what he referred to as "the civic coefficients of our intellectual passions" (Polanyi 1958, 217).

For Polanyi, there was an important relationship between knowledge and organization; moreover, this relationship was one that should be culti- vated and preserved as the wellspring of creativity. Within this view, diver- sity and locality are necessarily integral to the scientific practice of individ- ual scientists. This is as true for multisite trials in Sri Lanka today as it was in the projects that Polanyi described. What we have tried to describe here are the nexuses that connect the "black box" of research activity (Hess 2001) with the wider social and political settings in which it is situated. Biomedi- cal research, particularly where multisite clinical trials are concerned, is car- ried out in diverse spaces and places, by people from a variety of social and cultural backgrounds. This variability adds a crucial element to Polanyi's postulation concerning power and structural injustice in scientific knowl- edge production. Key to this move for us has been a focus on collaboration across multiple lines of difference.

Throughout this work, we have treated collaboration as an emic concept, a term deployed widely to capture rhetorically the kind of relationships to which people aspire when they work together on joint research projects. We have paid attention not just to the senior researchers and why they collaborate (Parker and Kingori 2016) but also to the junior and midlevel researchers so that we can map out what they gain from being part of global research networks. In the context of cross-cultural collaborations, we extend Strathern's notion that collaboration is not merely a *practice* but also operates as a *value* (Strathern 2011). As we argued in chapter 4, it is also a value that carries with it *potentiality*, in that it is at once strategic, forward-looking, and aspirational. Crucially, the move brings into focus the way that trialists, both Sri Lankan and expatriate, are able to use, often in ingenious ways, the human, intellectual, and material resources that are to hand to realize the *potentiality* of collaboration. For these reasons, collaboration resonates strongly with the idea of development. In making a switch from the external form of clinical trials to their internal relations, we have been able to bring into focus the way that social and political values are reconfigured in the face of expert systems that originate in faraway places.

This view of collaboration foregrounds local researchers as active and creative participants in the exchange that is taking place. They are not simply on the receiving end in a hub-and-spoke model of biomedical research activity. Nor are they caught in a double-bind of gratitude and resentment—that is, reliant on and thankful for the attentions of the global north (for example, when in receipt of funding, infrastructure, personnel, or expert knowledge), yet resentful that this is always on and in another's terms. In fact, there is no simple submission to the rationality of the randomized controlled trial (RCT) at all; crucially, we see evidence of conflict and creativity when it comes to making things work. The Sri Lankan collaborators we have introduced in this book were thus not mere recipients of external research activity and the development possibilities it might bring. The versions of the development processes they articulated to us revealed attempts to actively shape the process to fit local circumstances. As part of this engagement, there are efforts to remoralize the relationship with distant counterparts, and there is no simple, passive acceptance of the material and intellectual assistance on offer. For their part, the Western researchers seek to gain competence in the norms and values of far-flung worlds, but the reverse move is equally important. Efforts to acquire what might be thought of as conceptual and collaborative fluency are in evidence when dealing with outside partners in the conduct of international trials.

With this countermove, novel and emergent geographies of international collaboration merge with old ones, bringing new configurations to scientific and technological sociality. Drawing ethnographic attention to the "doing" rather than the "being done to" takes us onto the next conceptual conjunction and a final reflection on the scope of bioethics.

Collaboration and Bioethics

In his critique of development, James Ferguson offered the notion of the "anti-politics machine" (Ferguson 1994). This image was meant to capture the ways in which development strategies, typically of the hub-and-spoke variety, proceed by suspending, obscuring, or defining as outside their scope the political concerns that are in fact central to those that the aid effort is intended to help. In the wake of development efforts, the effect of the machine is to extend bureaucratic state power in line with external interests. Essential to the anti-politics machine, Ferguson argued, is the "less-developed country" as a foundational construction. We would suggest that in the account we have developed here there are some useful parallels to be drawn with the way in which bioethics operates within the context of biomedical research collaborations.

There is a similar definition of focus in which international interests are cast as inherently benevolent—but in ways that leave the broader political context of trialing and experimentation outside its scope. Regulatory frameworks, such as those available in the form of ICH-GCP guidelines, need to be in place for "ethical" research to happen. However, bioethics as it operates through a variety of practices and discourses is in its own way an anti-politics machine, recasting and thereby containing political questions as ethical ones. Likewise, there is, somewhere in the background, the construction of the "less-ethical country," one that needs to be educated and brought into line with regard to the practice of bioethics, which continually emerges as a deficient capacity. There is, in short, an incommensurability between the reach of bioethics as this is actualized as part of the assemblage of the multi-site clinical trial on the one hand and, on the other, the landscape of political interests and concerns as they existed in Sri Lanka at the time of our research. In the changing relationship between markets, development, and new scientific knowledge in the global south, what is encompassed and acted upon in the name of morality, humanism, justice, and, the case in point here, bioethics does not map straightforwardly onto local specificities. The exchanges documented in chapter 8 revealed the practical and conceptual messiness of managing this incommensurability. They illuminated different articulations of power and the points of friction that arise when these are brought together.

This move takes us away from the hub-and-spoke model of how ideas and practices are diffused globally, and we step into the more complex and conflicted flow of concepts and resources that are needed to make a trial happen outside the global north. In this flow are mixed desires that may not sit comfortably together: the protection of local populations may be one group's primary objective whereas the facilitation of clinical trials may be another's. As we saw in chapter 8, the normative systems governing research ethics are ambivalent and contested, and they play into wider conflicts in which the notion of ethics might be used strategically to bring about desired ends outside of the trial per se. Such systems operate rather like the semiotician's floating signifier—that is, they convey a greater sense of their concreteness than the things that they reference and are therefore capable of carrying multiple contradictions.

Of relevance to the kind of analysis we have been trying to develop within this book, these contradictions do not only figure in the discourses of our interlocutors. We ourselves have struggled with questions of what makes trial activity ethical or unethical. We did not work in these trials in any sense as normative bioethicists, and neither did we set out to answer this question in quite the way a bioethicist would, but we also acknowledge that there are no "moral exteriorities" in a study such as this (Biruk 2017; Fassin 2008). The collaborative ethnography we have undertaken situates us within the communities we studied, so our end point cannot be any simple meta-wisdom distilled from the field of conflicts and contradictions in which we found ourselves. An ethnographic attention to detail begins to highlight how, within such a complex assemblage, our engagement made different significations become visible. By focusing on the way two different kinds of trials were set up and run—one for a joint pain treatment and the other for an antidote to paraquat—we go beyond scientific questions and the normative ethics that govern them.

Our approach brings into view a wider field of ethical concerns such as the role of funders, access to medicines, choices of collaborative partners, engagement with local regulatory infrastructures, and levels of health care provision locally. In this framing, ethics is emergent rather than given, a matter of politics rather than rule-based governance, and a feature of structural inequality rather than cultural diversity. Whereas bioethics might operate as an anti-politics machine, the practice of collaboration appears to work in the opposite direction by rendering the parameters of bioethics potent, porous, and open to revision and reinterpretation. One of our main contributions to ongoing discussions regarding the place of biomedical research within global projects of progress, modernization, and development has thus been to place those directly involved with effecting change back at the center of the analysis. Whereas the machine metaphor is apt to marginalize the movers and shakers in the clinical trials assemblage, we have tried to give them voice and to understand their motivations.

It has been our intention to describe from the ground up the rhetorics that are involved in getting one version of what is the ethical way to proceed to predominate over another. Reintroducing the actors who are often invisible—and drawing attention to the wrinkles and creases that are rendered flat, featureless, and peripheral in the global gaze of bioethics—is an important step because it takes us beyond the formality of ethical guidelines and their role in regulating research practice (described earlier) and into the tacit, day-to-day social relations that enable research processes to proceed in the first place (also as described earlier). In contemplating the relationship between collaboration and bioethics, we are thus extending ideas of what bioethics "does" to encompass a situated research ethics with collaboration at its core. This tactic looks beyond the normative framework of international collaborative research and reveals new and unexpected ways in which research operates as a form of development praxis that can transfigure relationships, values, and ethics into something that they were not in the past. Change is incremental and disparate in its consequences rather than revolutionary and causally linear.

In our attempts to characterize these processes, we have considered unintended consequences as well as intended ones. An image that has helped in this is that of the rhizome (cf. Choy et al. 2009). Unlike other images, this one suggests unpredictable and irregular formations rather than predetermined structures of growth and development. In this instance, local stipulations (made by the ethics committee) combined with the changing fortunes and strategic interests of the multinational company behind the Joint Pain

Trial meant that the excursion into clinical trials as a commercial venture never materialized. Lanka Trials failed to take off as a vehicle for global clinical trials. The expected narrative was one of success guaranteed by the backing of powerful multinational pharmaceutical interests rather than one of failure. Equally, the Paraquat Poisoning Trial did not show efficacy in reducing mortality and might also have been thought to be a failure. That said, it is commonplace for trials to fail, and this does not mean they were done badly or were in some sense "wrong." As Ferguson commented when speaking of development, "what may be the most important about a development project is not so much what it does do but what it fails to do; it may be that its real importance in the end lies in the 'side effects'" (Ferguson 1994, 254).

Both trials failed to bring positive results in the pharmaceutical sense, but the more important point that we want to make is that changes in the sector of clinical research did occur, albeit not in the ways envisaged! In both instances, considerable capacity was built in terms of training, infrastructure, and the conceptual knowledge needed to conduct a multisite RCT. To return to the cargo-cult analogy presented in chapter 6, the landing strip was carefully built by the local researchers even if the cargo never came. In each of the trials we followed, potentiality was never actualized in the ways that were predicted. Yet they were, in many respects, very successful failures. In terms of first-order development, they built human resources locally, inducted new recruits into the research assemblage, and created visibility for Sri Lankan researchers as motivated and capable of doing such research. It also embedded researchers from outside Sri Lanka into the local networks in new ways— as is evident, for example, in the evolution of the South Asian Clinical Toxicology Research Collaboration (SACTRC) beyond the period followed in this study. The Paraquat Poisoning Trial might not have shown efficacy in reducing mortality, but participants in the study did do better than those who were not involved due to the closer care that they received; the study also trained several junior researchers, who became doctors who understood poisoning patients a little better; and the results persuaded agricultural policy makers to remove paraquat from the market. In second-order terms, the trials introduced and embedded conceptual shifts in practice and policy in relation to local thinking about the nature of human subject research, as discussed in chapter 5.

From the perspective of research on clinical trials and collaboration, these are developments that took place over a considerable period of time. A shallow reading of clinical trials activity takes a view that sees researchers merely slicing into networks of connection for the duration of one trial. In so doing, such studies fail to account for how change takes place and why, and how there might be outcomes that cannot be second-guessed. The approach we have taken here reveals that "capacity" is not simply absent, as in the hub-and-spoke model, but present in multiple forms, which lead to development outcomes that are diverse and often unintended. After the trials have left town, many things are not quite as they were before.

NOTES

1. International Collaborative Research in Biomedicine

1. The International Science and Bioethics Collaborations project was funded by the U.K. Economic and Social Research Council (ESRC) grant number RES-062-23-0215. The project included ten anthropology researchers from Cambridge University, Durham University, and Sussex University. Along with Sri Lanka, the researchers focused on India, the People's Republic of China, Taiwan, and South Korea, investigating international collaborations and stem cell research.

2. The authors are introduced using their full names but thereafter will be referred to by their first name only. All other individuals who participated in the research are identified by their roles only to preserve their anonymity. We shared drafts of this book with the key research participants at various stages in its development.

3. "Collaboration" in *Collins English Dictionary* (Glasgow: HarperCollins, 2018), https://www.collinsdictionary.com/dictionary/english/collaboration.

2. Collaboration in Context

1. For example, see the details of the World Bank's project "Sri Lanka: Health Sector Development" (Project ID: P050740, approval date: 2004; closing date: 2010), http://projects.worldbank.org/P050740/health-sector-development?lang=en.

2. Notwithstanding these trends, Sri Lanka is often cited as a nation that has been able to achieve improvements in the health of its population that are disproportionate to the state of the county's economy (Nuffield Council on Bioethics 2002, 20). With health expenditures running at only 3 percent of the gross domestic product (compared with 7.1 percent in Japan, and 5.2 percent in India), Sri Lanka still maintains a comparatively high level of life expectancy for the region (65 years for men and 73 years for women), and it also maintains a relatively high ratio of doctors and nurses to the general population (36.5 doctors and 102.7 nurses per 100,000 of the population).

3. For example, Buddha is often compared to a physician diagnosing an illness and prescribing its cure. As the influential scholar-priest Walpola Rahula pointed out, "he is the wise and scientific doctor of the world [*Bhisakka* or *Bhaiṣajya-guru*]" (Rahula 1978, 17).

4. See the Institute for Research and Development's site at http://www.ird.lk/.

5. See NASTEC (2003). Also see the subsequent guidelines produced in the field of assisted reproductive technology (https://web.archive.org/web/20090604211953/http://www.slmedc.lk/publications/AssistedReproductiveTechnologies.htm).

6. See, for example, the International Collaboration Awards, an initiative launched by the U.K. Royal Society to promote international collaborative research (https://royalsociety.org/grants-schemes-awards/grants/international-collaborations/). Also see the Royal Society's 2017 report on a survey of international collaboration and mobility, which shows a marked increase in such activity.

7. The meeting took place at King's College, London, in September 2009.

8. ELSI first appeared as part of the work of the National Human Genome Research Institute (NHGRI) and was established in 1990 as an integral part of the Human Genome Project (HGP).

3. The Joint Pain Trial

1. Clinical trials are experiments designed to evaluate drugs, devices, or medical procedures. Trials aim to produce replicable data about the effectiveness of different interventions before they are made available for commercial or other use. According to the WHO guidelines, there are normally four phases through which new chemical compounds must progress (WHO 1995). From one stage to the next, the dosage of the drugs and the number of people exposed to the drug are gradually increased. Phase 1 clinical trials, otherwise known as "first in-human trials," are performed using healthy individuals to identify preliminary evidence of safety. Phases 2 to 4 are often performed with patients who have the condition for which the drug is intended. Studies to reproduce drugs that are out of patent and have already been tested (so-called generics) use primarily healthy individuals to measure the absorption and efficacy of the tested drug as compared with an existing

one. Trials can also be performed on existing medicines approved for a new condition, to validate an existing clinical practice for which there is some evidence but not yet proved with an RCT, or in an attempt to find more effective combinations. Trials also can be conducted using new populations to access new markets. Finally, pharmaceutical companies also use trials to extend their patents by creating new formulas (for example, developing a drug in liquid rather than tablet form) to ensure a monopoly for the product and thereby avoid the risk of losing its patent to cheaper alternatives.

5. Localizing Ethics

1. We are grateful to Claudia Merli for pointing out an earlier genealogy of this distinction that goes back to Heidegger, whose notion of being-in-the-world (*dasein*) was built on the idea of caring for others.

6. Negotiating Collaborative Research

1. Cargo cults was the term used to describe millenarian movements that sprang up across Papua New Guinea in the wake of contact with Westerners. Fascinated by the goods they brought ["cargo"], the people began to create conditions that would facilitate the arrival of future wealth and prosperity, such as making landing strips to encourage the arrival of aeroplanes (Burridge 1969).

7. Precarious Ethics

1. We do not wish to invoke the whole of Kristeva's psychoanalytic project in the context of Sri Lankan society, but her conceptualization of the "abject" as being neither object nor subject has been helpful in developing the argument we put forward here.

2. Decontamination of the stomach was often spoken of as gastric lavage and/or forced emesis. In practice this usually meant making patients drink water mixed with sodium bicarbonate to induce vomiting. Patients might also be subject to flushing the stomach with water *or* given activated charcoal *or* a combination of all of these. Despite the fact that the concepts were collapsed together like this, different practices have differing consequences on the patients' conditions—for example, vomiting with sodium bicarbonate is not recommended in international toxicology guidelines as it may tear the digestive track and actually make the toxins absorb faster. Therefore, clarity on what the clinical practice is, and should be, matters for the recovery of the patient.

8. Strategic Ethics

1. A contributor from Pakistan planned to attend but unfortunately had to cancel at the last minute due to family reasons.

2. Institute of Research and Development (http://www.ird.lk).

3. "Death of Patient in Kurunegala Hospital," *Lakbima*, January 27, 2003. See also "Poisoned Patient in Critical Condition Dies Due to an Experimental Charcoal Treatment," *Lanka Deepa*, January 28, 2003.

4. "More on 'Poison Plant Fuels Suicide,'" *The Island* [Online Edition], April 17, 2006, http://www.island.lk/2006/04/17/opinion5.html.

BIBLIOGRAPHY

Abeykoon, Palitha T. P. L. 1998. *Population and Manpower Resources of Sri Lanka*. Colombo, Sri Lanka: Natural Resources, Energy, and Science Authority.

——. 2003. "The Implications of Technology Change for Health Care Delivery in Sri Lanka." Colombo, Sri Lanka: World Health Organization. http://citeseerx.ist.psu.edu /viewdoc/download?doi=10.1.1.604.1118&rep=rep1&type=pdf.

Abraham, Itty. 2006. "The Contradictory Spaces of Postcolonial Techno-Science." *Economic and Political Weekly* 41 (3): 210–17. http://www.jstor.org/stable/4417699

Abraham, John. 2007. "Drug trials and evidence bases in international regulatory context." *BioSocieties*. 2 (1): 41–56.

Abraham, John, and Tim Reed. 2002. "Progress, Innovation and Regulatory Science in Drug Development: The Politics of International Standard-Setting." *Social Studies of Science* 32 (3): 337–69. https://doi.org/10.1177/0306312702032003001.

Adams, V., S. Miller, S. Craig, Nyima, Sonam, Droyoung, Lhakpen, M. Varner. 2005. "The Challenge of Cross-Cultural Clinical Trials Research: Case Report from the Tibetan Autonomous Region, People's Republic of China." *Medical Anthropology* 19 (3): 267–89. http://www.jstor.org/stable/3655363.

Agamben, Giorgio. 1998. *Homo Sacer: Sovereign Power and Bare Life*. Stanford, CA: Stanford University Press.

Akrong, Lloyd, Klasien Horstman, and Daniel K. Arhinful. 2014. "Informed Consent and Clinical Trial Participation: Perspectives from a Ghanaian Community." In *Making Global Health Care Innovation Work*, edited by Nora Engel, Ine Van Hoyweghen, and Anja Krumeich, 17–39. New York: Palgrave Macmillan. https://doi.org/10.1057/9781137456038_2.

Allden, K., L. Jones, I Weissbecker, M. Wessells, P. Bolton, T. S. Betancourt, Z. Hijazi, et al. 2009. "Mental Health and Psychosocial Support in Crisis and Conflict: Report of the Mental Health Working Group." In "2009 Humanitarian Action Summit," edited by Frederick M. Burkle and Michael VanRooyen, Supplement. *Prehospital and Disaster Medicine* 24 (Suppl. 2): S217–27. https://doi.org/10.1017/S1049023X00021622.

Aluwihare, A. P. R. 1982. "Traditional and Western Medicine Working in Tandem." *World Health Forum* 3 (4): 450–51.

Anderson, M. S., and N. H. Steneck, eds. 2011. *International Research Collaborations: Much to Be Gained, Many Ways to Get in Trouble*. London: Routledge.

Anderson, Warwick. 2002. Introduction: Postcolonial Technoscience. *Social Studies of Science* 32 (5/6): 643–658.

——. 2008. *The Collectors of Lost Souls: Turning Kuru Scientists into Whitemen*. Baltimore: Johns Hopkins University Press.

——. 2009. "From Subjugated Knowledge to Conjugated Subjects: Science and Globalisation, or Postcolonial Studies of Science?" *Postcolonial Studies* 12 (4): 389–400. https://doi.org/10.1080/13688790903350641.

Angell, Marcia. 1997. "The Ethics of Clinical Research in the Third World." *New England Journal of Medicine* 337: 847–56. https://doi.org/10.1056/NEJM199709183371209.

Appadurai, Arjun. 2000. "Grassroots Globalization and the Research Imagination." *Public Culture* 12 (1): 1–19. http://muse.jhu.edu/journals/public_culture/v012/12.1appadurai.html.

Arnold, David. 2000. *Science, Technology and Medicine in Colonial India*. Cambridge: Cambridge University Press.

Arseculeratne, S. N. 1999. "The Determinants of the Growth of Science in Pre-Modern South Asia." In *History and Politics: Millennial Perspectives. Essays in Honour of Kingsley de Silva*, edited by G. Peiris and S. W. R. A. De Samarasinghe, 289–306. Colombo, Sri Lanka: Law & Society Trust.

——. 2008. "What Constitutes the Enterprise of Modern Science?" *Journal of the National Science Foundation of Sri Lanka* 34 (4): 257–66.

——. 2010. *Education in medicine as a component of modern science: Restoring the balance*. Paper presented at the IMEC 2010 conference "The Future of Medical Education" at the International Medical University, Kuala Lumpur, Malaysia, March 24–26.

Atkinson, Sarah. 2016. "Care, Kidneys and Clones: The Distance of Space, Time and Imagination." In *The Edinburgh Companion to the Critical Medical Humanities*, edited by A. Whitehead and A. Woods, 611–26. Edinburgh: Edinburgh University Press.

Balmer, Andrew S., Jane Calvert, Claire Marris, Susan Molyneux-Hodgson, Emma Frow, Matthew Kearnes, Kate Bulpin, Pablo Schyfter, Adrian MacKenzie, and Paul Martin. 2015. "Taking Roles in Interdisciplinary Collaborations: Reflections on Working in Post-ELSI Spaces in the UK Synthetic Biology Community." *Science and Technology Studies* 28 (3): 3–25. http://ojs.tsv.fi/index.php/sts/article/view/55340.

Beauchamp, Tom L., and James F. Childress. 1989. *Principles of Biomedical Ethics*. 3rd ed. New York: Oxford University Press.

Beaver, Donald, and R. Rosen. 1978. "Studies in Scientific Collaboration. Part I: The Professional Origins of Scientific Co-Authorship." *Scientometrics* 1 (1): 65–84. https://doi.org/10.1007/BF02016840.

———. 1979a. "Studies in Scientific Collaboration. Part II: Scientific Co-Authorship, Research Productivity and Visibility in the French Scientific Elite, 1799–1830." *Scientometrics* 1 (2): 133–49. https://doi.org/10.1007/BF02016966.

———. 1979b. "Studies in Scientific Collaboration Part III. Professionalization and the Natural History of Modern Scientific Co-Authorship." *Scientometrics* 1 (3): 231–45. https://doi.org/10.1007/BF02016308.

Beisel, Uli. 2015. "The Blue Warriors: Ecology, Participation and Public Health in Malaria Control Experiments." In *Para-States and Medical Science: Making African Global Health*, edited by P. Wenzel Geissler, 281–303. Durham, NC: Duke University Press.

Bell, Susan E., and Anne E. Figert. 2012. "Medicalization and Pharmaceuticalization at the Intersections: Looking Backward, Sideways and Forward." *Social Science and Medicine* 75 (5): 775–83. https://doi.org/10.1016/j.socscimed.2012.04.002.

Benatar, Solomon R. 2002. "Reflections and Recommendations on Research Ethics in Developing Countries." *Social Science and Medicine* 54 (7): 1131–41. http://hdl.handle.net/10822/1011246.

Benatar, S. R., A. S. Daar, and P. A. Singer. 2005. "Global Health Challenges: The Need for an Expanded Discourse on Bioethics." *PLoS Med* 2 (7): e143. https://doi.org/10.1371/journal.pmed.0020143.

Beran, David, Peter Byass, Aiah Gbakima, Kathleen Kahn, Osman Sankoh, Stephen Tollman, Miles Witham, and Justine Davies. 2017. "Research Capacity Building—Obligations for Global Health Partners." *Lancet Global Health* 5 (6): e567–68. https://doi.org/10.1016/S2214-109X(17)30180-8.

Bhattacharya, Sanjoy. 2006. *Expunging Variola : The Control and Eradication of Smallpox in India, 1947–1977*. Hyderabad, India: Orient Longman.

Bhutta, Zulfiqar, Samiran Nundy, and Kamran Abbasi. 2004. "Is There Hope for South Asia?" (Editorial.) *BMJ* 328: 777 https://doi.org/10.1136/bmj.328.7443.777.

Biehl, João G. 2004. "The Activist State: Global Pharmaceuticals, AIDS, and Citizenship in Brazil." *Social Text* 22 (3): 105–32. http://muse.jhu.edu/journals/soc/summary/v022/22.3biehl.html.

———. 2007. "Pharmaceuticalization: AIDS Treatment and Global Health Politics." *Anthropological Quarterly* 80 (4): 1083–126. https://doi.org/10.1353/anq.2007.0056.

Biehl, João G., B. Good, and A. Kleinman, eds. 2007. *Subjectivity: Ethnographic Investigations*. Berkeley: University of California Press.

Biehl, João G., and Adriana Petryna, eds. 2013. *When People Come First: Critical Studies in Global Health*. Princeton, NJ: Princeton University Press.

Biruk, Crystal. 2012. "Seeing Like a Research Project: Producing 'High-Quality Data' in AIDS Research in Malawi." *Medical Anthropology* 31 (4): 347–66. https://doi.org/10.1080/01459740.2011.631960.

———. 2017. "Ethical Gifts? An Analysis of Soap-for-Data Transactions in Malawian Survey Research Worlds." *Medical Anthropology Quarterly* 31 (3): 365–84. https://doi.org/10.1111/maq.12374.

Bloch, M. 2008. "Truth and Sight: Generalizing without Universalizing." *Journal of the Royal Anthropological Institute* 14 (Suppl. 1): S22–32. https://doi.org/0.1111/j.1467-9655.2008.00490.x.

Bolz, Waltraud. 2002. "Psychological Analysis of the Sri Lankan Conflict Culture with Special Reference to the High Suicide Rate." *Crisis* 23 (4): 167–70. https://doi.org/10.1027//0227-5910.23.4.167.

Boulding, Harriet. 2017. "Capacity Building as Instrument and Empowerment: Training Health Workers for Community-Based Roles in Ghana." *Cambridge Anthropology* 35 (1): 84–98.

Bourdieu, Pierre. 1993. *The Field of Cultural Production: Essays on Art and Literature.* Cambridge: Polity Press.

Boyer, D. 2008. "Thinking through the Anthropology of Experts." *Anthropology in Action* 15 (2): 38–46. https://doi.org/10.3167/aia.2008.150204.

Bracanovic, Tomislav. 2013. "Against Culturally Sensitive Bioethics." *Medicine, Health Care and Philosophy* 16 (4): 647–52. https://doi.org/10.1007/s11019-013-9504-2.

Brives, Charlotte. 2013. "Identifying Ontologies in a Clinical Trial." *Social Studies of Science* 43 (3): 397–416. https://doi.org/10.1177/0306312712472406.

———. 2016. "Biomedical Packages: Adjusting Drug, Bodies, and Environment in a Phase III Clinical Trial." *Medicine Anthropology Theory* 3 (1): 1–28.

Brown, Hannah. 2015. "Global Health Partnerships, Governance, and Sovereign Responsibility in Western Kenya." *American Ethnologist* 42 (2): 340–55. https://doi.org/10.1111/amet.12134.

Brown, Hannah, and Maia Green. 2015. "At the Service of Community Development: The Professionalization of Volunteer Work in Kenya and Tanzania." *African Studies Review* 58 (2): 63–84. https://doi.org/10.1017/asr.2015.38.

Bruun Jensen, Casper, and Wintherreik, Brit Ross. 2013. *Monitoring Movements in Development Aid: Recursive Partnerships and Infrastructures.* Cambridge, MA: MIT Press.

Buckley, Nicholas A., Lakshman Karalliedde, Andrew Dawson, Nimal Senanayake, and Michael Eddleston. 2004. "Where Is the Evidence for Treatments Used in Pesticide Poisoning? Is Clinical Toxicology Fiddling While the Developing World Burns?" *Clinical Toxicology* 42 (1): 113–16. https://doi.org/10.1081/CLT-120028756.

Burridge, K. 1969. *New Heaven, New Earth: A Study of Millenarian Activities.* London: Basil Blackwell.

Buruma, I., and A. Margalit. 2005. *Occidentalism: The West in the Eyes of Its Enemies.* Harmondsworth, United Kingdom: Penguin.

Cambrosio, A., P. Keating, T. Schlich, and G. Weisz. 2006. "Regulatory Objectivity and the Generation and Management of Evidence in Medicine." *Social Science and Medicine* 63 (1): 189–99. https://doi.org/10.1016/j.socscimed.2005.12.007.

Campbell, A. V. 2000. "'My Country Tis of Thee'—the Myopia of American Bioethics." *Medicine, Health Care and Philosophy* 3 (2): 195–98. https://doi.org/10.1023/A:1009907314602.

Carrier, J. G. 1995. *Occidentalism: Images of the West.* Oxford: Clarendon Press.

Carrithers, Michael. 1985. "An Alternative Social History of the Self." In *The Category of the Person: Anthropology, Philosophy and History*, edited by Michael Carrithers, Steven Collins, and Steven Lukes, 234–56. Cambridge: Cambridge University Press.

Chapin, Bambi L. 2014. *Childhood in a Sri Lankan Village: Shaping Hierarchy and Desire.* New Brunswick, NJ: Rutgers University Press.

Chataway, Joanna, Dinar Kale, and David Wield. 2007. "The Indian Pharmaceutical Industry before and after TRIPS." *Technology Analysis and Strategic Management* 19 (5): 559–63. https://doi.org/10.1080/09537320701521267.

Chattopadhyay, Subrata, and Raymond De Vries. 2008. "Bioethical Concerns Are Global, Bioethics Is Western." *Eubios Journal of Asian and International Bioethics* 18 (4): 106–9. https://www.ncbi.nlm.nih.gov/pmc/articles/PMC2707840/.

———. 2013. "Respect for Cultural Diversity in Bioethics Is an Ethical Imperative." *Medicine, Health Care, and Philosophy* 16 (4): 639–45. https://doi.org/10.1007/s11019-012-9433-5.

Chilisa, Bagele. 2005. "Educational Research within Postcolonial Africa: A Critique of HIV/AIDS Research in Botswana." *International Journal of Qualitative Studies in Education* 18 (6): 659–84. https://doi.org/10.1080/09518390500298170.

Chin, J. J. 2002. "Doctor-Patient Relationship: From Medical Paternalism to Enhanced Autonomy." *Singapore Medical Journal* 43 (3): 152–55.

Choy, Timothy K., Lieba Faier, Michael J. Hathaway, Miyako Inoue, Shiho Satsuka, and Anna Tsing. 2009. "A New Form of Collaboration in Cultural Anthropology: Matsutake Worlds." *American Ethnologist* 36 (2): 380–403. https://doi.org/10.1111/j.1548-1425.2009.01141.x.

Clifford, J., and George E. Marcus, eds. 1986. *Writing Culture: The Poetics and Politics of Ethnography*. Berkeley: University of California Press.

Collins, H. 2014. "Rejecting Knowledge Claims inside and outside Science." *Social Studies of Science* 44 (5): 722–35. https://doi.org/10.1177/0306312714536011.

Commission on Health Research for Development (COHRED). 1990. *Health Research: Essential Link to Equity and Development.* Oxford: Oxford University Press.

Cooper, Melinda. 2011. "Experimental Republic: Medical Accidents (Productive and Unproductive) in Postsocialist China." *East Asian Science, Technology and Society* 5 (3): 313–27. https://doi.org/10.1215/18752160-1407924.

———. 2013. "Double Exposure-Sex Workers, Biomedical Prevention Trials, and the Dual Logic of Global Public Health." *Scholar and Feminist Online* 11 (3): 1–11. http://sfonline.barnard.edu/life-un-ltd-feminism-bioscience-race/double-exposure-sex-workers-biomedical-prevention-trials-and-the-dual-logic-of-global-public-health/.

Cooper, Melinda, and Catherine Waldby. 2014. *Clinical Labor: Human Research Subjects and Tissue Donors in the Global Bioeconomy.* Durham, NC: Duke University Press.

Cooray, Prasanna. 2016. "Senaka Bibile: The God of Small Things." *Sri Lanka Guardian*, September 23. https://www.slguardian.org/senaka-bibilethe-god-of-small-things/.

Corsín Jiménez, Alberto. 2011. "Trust in Anthropology." *Anthropological Theory* 11 (2): 177–96. https://doi.org/10.1177/1463499611407392.

Council for International Organizations of Medical Sciences (CIOMS). 2016. *International Ethical Guidelines for Health-related Research Involving Humans.* 4th ed. Geneva: Council for International Organizations of Medical Sciences.

Crane, Johanna T. 2013. *Scrambling for Africa: AIDS, Expertise, and the Rise of American Global Health Science*. Ithaca, NY: Cornell University Press.

Daniel, E. V. 1984. *Fluid Signs: Being a Person the Tamil Way*. Berkeley: University of California Press.

———. 1989. "The Semeiosis of Suicide in Sri Lanka." In *Semiotics, Self, and Society*, edited by B Lee and G Urban, 69–100. Berlin: Mouton de Gruyter.

Das, V., and R. K. Das. 2007. "How the Body Speaks: Illness and the Lifeworld among the Urban Poor." In *Subjectivity: Ethnographic Investigations.*, edited by João G. Biehl, B. Good, and A. Kleinman, 66–97. Berkeley: University of California Press.

Daston, Lorraine, and Peter Galison. 2007. *Objectivity*. New York: Zone Books.

Davis, A. M., S. C. Hull, and C. Grady. 2002. "The Invisible Hand in Clinical Research: The Study Coordinator's Critical Role in Human Subject Protection." *Journal of Law, Medicine and Ethics* 30: 411–19. https://doi.org/10.1111/j.1748-720X.2002.tb00410.x.

Dawson, A., and N. Buckley. 2007. "Integrating Approaches to Paraquat Poisoning." *Ceylon Medical Journal* 52 (2): 45–47. https://doi.org/10.4038/cmj.v52i2.1018.

De Alwis, Malathi. 2012. "'Girl Still Burning inside My Head': Reflections on Suicide in Sri Lanka." *Contributions to Indian Sociology* 46 (1–2): 29–51. https://doi.org/10.1177/006996671104600203.

Decoteau, C. 2013. *Ancestors and Antiretrovirals: The Bio-Politics of HIV/AIDS in Post-Apartheid South Africa*. Chicago: University of Chicago Press.

De Silva, H. A., M. M. D. Fonseka, A. Pathmeswaran, D. G. S. Alahakone, G. A. Ratnatilake, S. B. Gunatilake, C. D. Ranasinha, D. G. Lalloo, J. K. Aronson, and H. J. de Silva. 2003. "Multiple-Dose Activated Charcoal for Treatment of Yellow Oleander Poisoning: A Single-Blind, Randomised, Placebo-Controlled Trial." *The Lancet* 361 (9373): 1935–38. https://doi.org/10.1016/S0140-6736(03)13581-7.

De Vries, P. 2007. "Don't Compromise Your Desire for Development! A Lacanian/Deleuzian Rethinking of the Anti-Politics Machine." *Third World Quarterly* 28 (1): 25–43. https://doi.org/10.1080/01436590601081765.

De Vries, Raymond. 2004. "How Can We Help? From 'Sociology in' to 'Sociology of' Bioethics." *Journal of Law, Medicine and Ethics* 32 (2): 279–92. https://doi.org/10.1111/j.1748-720X.2004.tb00475.x.

De Vries, Raymond, Leslie M. Rott, and Yasaswi Paruchuri. 2011. "Normative Environments of International Science." In *International Research Collaborations: Much to Be Gained, Many Ways to Get in Trouble*, edited by Melissa S. Anderson and Nicholas H. Steneck, 105–20. London: Taylor & Francis. https://doi.org/10.4324/9780203848906.

Deleuze, Gilles, and Félix Guattari. 1987. *A Thousand Plateaus: Capitalism and Schizophrenia*. Minneapolis: University of Minnesota Press.

Deshapriya, S., and A. Welikala. 2004. "Paradise Lost." *Index on Censorship* 33 (4): 190–94. https://doi.org/10.1080/03064220408537422.

Deshpande, R. S. 2002. "Suicide by Farmers in Karnataka: Agrarian Distress and Possible Alleviatory Steps." *Economic and Political Weekly* 37 (26): 2601–10. http://www.jstor.org/stable/4412301.

Dilley, Roy. 2010. "Reflections on Knowledge Practices and the Problem of Ignorance." In "Making Knowledge," edited by Trevor H. J. Marchand, Supplement. *Journal of the Royal Anthropological Institute* 16 (Suppl. 1): S176–92. https://doi.org/10.1111/j.1467 -9655.2010.01616.x.

Dissanayake, Vajira H. W., N. Mendis, and R. D. Lanerolle. 2006. "Research Ethics and Ethical Review Committees in Sri Lanka: A 25 Year Journey." *Ceylon Medical Journal* 51 (3): 110–13. http://doi.org/10.4038/cmj.v51i3.1254.

Dixon, J. R. 1998. "The International Conference on Harmonization Good Clinical Practice Guideline." *Quality Assurance* 6 (2): 65–74.

Dixon, Justin. 2017. "Disease, Morality and Bioethics: An Ethnographic Study of a TB Vaccine Trial Site in South Africa." PhD diss., Durham University.

Douglas-Jones, Rachel. 2012. "Locating Ethics: Capacity Building, Ethics Review and Research Governance across Asia." PhD diss., Durham University. http://etheses.dur .ac.uk/6970/.

Douglas-Jones, Rachel. 2017. "Building Capacity in Ethical Review: Compliance and Transformation in the Asia-Pacific Region." *Cambridge Anthropology* 35 (1): 49–66.

Douglas-Jones, Rachel, and Salla Sariola. 2009. "Rhizome Yourself: Experiencing Deleuze and Guattari from Theory to Practice." *Rhizomes* 19 (Summer). http://www.rhizomes .net/issue19/sariola.html.

Douglas-Jones, Rachel, and Justin Shaffner. 2017. "Hope and Insufficiency: Capacity Building in Ethnographic Comparison." *Cambridge Anthropology* 35 (1): 1–16.

Duffield, Mark. 2002. "Social Reconstruction and the Radicalization of Development: Aid as a Relation of Global Liberal Governance." *Development and Change* 33 (5): 1049–71. https://doi.org/10.1111/1467-7660.t01-1-00260.

Dumit, Joseph. 2012. *Drugs for Life: How Pharmaceutical Companies Define Our Health.* Durham: Duke University Press.

Dumont, L. 1970. *Homo Hierarchicus: The Caste System and Its Implications.* London: Weidenfeld & Nicholson.

Durante, C. 2009. "Bioethics in a Pluralistic Society: Bioethical Methodology in Lieu of Moral Diversity." *Medicine, Health Care and Philosophy* 12: 37–47. https://doi.org/10 .1007/s11019-008-9148-9.

Dutta, Achintya Kumar. 2008. "Pursuit of Medical Knowledge: Charles Donovan (1863– 1951) on Kala-Azar in India." *Journal of Medical Biography* 16 (2): 72–76. https://doi .org/10.1258/jmb.2007.007004.

Ebrahimnejad, Hormoz, ed. 2009. *The Development of Modern Medicine in Non-Western Countries: Historical Perspectives.* London: Routledge..

Ecks, Stefan. 2005. "Pharmaceutical Citizenship: Antidepressant Marketing and the Promise of Demarginalization in India." *Anthropology and Medicine* 12 (3): 239–54. https://doi.org/10.1080/13648470500291360.

Eddleston, Michael, C. A. Ariaratnam, W. P. Meyer, G. Perera, A. M. Kularatne, S. Attapattu, M. H. R. Sheriff, and D. A. Warrell. 1999. "Epidemic of Self-Poisoning with Seeds of the Yellow Oleander Tree (*Thevetia peruviana*) in Northern Sri Lanka." *Tropical Medicine and International Health* 4 (4): 266–73. https://doi.org/10.1046/j.1365 -3156.1999.00397.x.

Eddleston, Michael, P. Eyer, and F. Worek. 2005. "Differences between Organophosphorus Insecticides in Human Self-Poisoning: A Prospective Cohort Study." *The Lancet* 366 (9495): 1452–59. https://doi.org/10.1016/S0140-6736(05)67598-8.

Eddleston, Michael, and S. Haggalla. 2007. "The Hazards of Gastric Lavage for Intentional Self-Poisoning in a Resource Poor Location." *Clinical Toxicology* 45: 136–43. https://doi.org/10.1080/15563650601006009.

Eddleston, Michael, Edmund Juszczak, Nick A. Buckley, Lalith Senarathna, Fahim Mohamed, Wasantha Dissanayake, Ariyasena Hittarage, et al. 2008. "Multiple-Dose Activated Charcoal in Acute Self-Poisoning: A Randomised Controlled Trial." *The Lancet* 371 (9612): 579–87. https://doi.org/10.1016/S0140-6736(08)60270-6.

Eddleston, Michael, S. Rajapakse, Rajakanthan, S. Jayalath, L. Sjöström, W. Santharaj, P. N. Thenabadu, M. H. R. Sheriff, and D. A. Warrell. 2000. "Anti-Digoxin Fab Fragments in Cardiotoxicity Induced by Ingestion of Yellow Oleander: A Randomised Controlled Trial." *The Lancet* 355 (9208): 967–72. https://doi.org/10.1016/S0140-6736(00)90014-X.

Eddleston, Michael, M. H. R. Sheriff, and K. Hawton. 1998. "Deliberate Self Harm in Sri Lanka: An Overlooked Tragedy in the Developing World." *BMJ* 317 (7151): 133–35. http://www.ncbi.nlm.nih.gov/pmc/articles/PMC1113497/.

Ekanayake, Samanthika, Martin Prince, Athula Sumathipala, Sisira Siribaddana, and Craig Morgan. 2013. "'We Lost All We Had in a Second': Coping with Grief and Loss after a Natural Disaster." *World Psychiatry* 12 (1): 69–75. https://doi.org/10.1002/wps.20018.

Elliott, Danielle, and Timothy K. Thomas. 2017. "Lost in Translation? On Collaboration between Anthropology and Epidemiology." *Medicine Anthropology Theory* 4 (2). https://doi.org/10.17157/mat.4.2.497.

Ellison, Susan. 2017. "Corrective Capacities: From Unruly Politics to Democratic Capacitacion." *Cambridge Anthropology* 35 (1): 67–83.

European Medicines Agency (EMA). 2012. "Reflection Paper on Ethical and GCP Aspects of Clinical Trials of Medicinal Products for Human Use Conducted outside of the EU/EEA and Submitted in Marketing-Authorisation Applications to the EU Regulatory Authorities." EMA/121340/2011, April 16. Working Group on Clinical Trials Conducted outside of the EU/EEA. http://www.ema.europa.eu/docs/en_GB/document_library/Regulatory_and_procedural_guideline/2012/04/WC500125437.pdf.

Emanuel, Ezekiel J., David Wendler, and Christine Grady. 2000. "What Makes Clinical Research Ethical?" *JAMA* 283 (20): 2701–11. https://doi.org/10.1001/jama.283.20.2701.

Emanuel, Ezekiel J., David Wendler, Jack Killen, and Christine Grady. 2004. "What Makes Clinical Research in Developing Countries Ethical? The Benchmarks of Ethical Research." *Journal of Infectious Diseases* 189 (5): 930–37. https://doi.org/10.1086/381709.

Englund, H., and J. Leach. 2000. "Ethnography and the Meta-Narratives of Modernity." *Current Anthropology* 41 (2): 225–48. http://www.jstor.org/stable/10.1086/300126.

Fallis, Don. 2006. "The Epistemic Costs and Benefits of Collaboration." *Southern Journal of Philosophy* 44 (Suppl. 1): 197–208. https://doi.org/10.1111/j.2041-6962.2006.tb00039.x.

Farmer, Paul. 1999. "Pathologies of Power: Rethinking Health and Human Rights." *American Journal of Public Health* 89 (10): 1486–96.https://doi.org/10.2105/AJPH.89.10.1486.

———. 2004. *Pathologies of Power: Health, Human Rights, and the New War on the Poor.* Vol. 22. Berkeley: University of California Press.

Fassin, Didier. 2008. "Beyond Good and Evil? Questioning the Anthropological Discomfort with Morals." *Anthropological Theory* 8 (4): 333–44.https://doi.org/10.1177/1463499608096642.

———. 2012. *Humanitarian Reason: A Moral History of the Present*. Berkeley: University of California Press.

Faubion, James D., and George E. Marcus. 2009. *Fieldwork Is Not What It Used to Be: Learning Anthropology's Method in a Time of Transition*. Ithaca, NY: Cornell University Press.

Ferguson, James. 1994. *The Anti-Politics Machine: "Development," Depoliticization, and Bureaucratic Power in Lesotho*. Minneapolis: University of Minnesota Press.

Fernando, Dulitha N. 2001. "Structural Adjustment Programmes and Healthcare Services in Sri Lanka: An Overview." In *Public Health and the Poverty of Reforms: The South Asian Predicament*, edited by Imrana Qadeer, Kasturi Sen, and K. R. Nayar, 311–26. London: Sage.

Fernando, R. 2007. "Management of Poisoning." Colombo, Sri Lanka: National Poisons Information Centre, National Hospital of Sri Lanka.

Feyerabend, P. 1999. *Conquest of Abundance: A Tale of Abstraction versus the Richness of Being*. Chicago: Chicago University Press.

Finkler, K. 2000. "Diffusion Reconsidered: Variation and Transformation in Biomedical Practice, a Case Study from Mexico." *Medical Anthropology* 19 (1): 1–39.https://doi.org/10.1080/01459740.2000.9966167.

Fisher, Jill. 2009. *Medical Research for Hire: The Political Economy of Pharmaceutical Clinical Trials*. New Brunswick, NJ: Rutgers University Press.

Fortun, K. 2001. *Advocacy after Bhopal: Environmentalism, Disaster, New Global Orders*. Chicago: Chicago University Press.

Foucault, Michel. 1978. *The History of Sexuality. Volume 1: An Introduction*. Translated by Robert Hurley. New York: Random House.

Fox, Renée C. 1990. "The Evolution of American Bioethics: A Sociological Perspective." In *Social Science Perspectives on Medical Ethics*, edited by G. Weisz, 201–20. Philadelphia: University of Pennsylvania Press. http://link.springer.com/chapter/10.1007/978-94-009-1930-3_11.

Gammelgaard, A. 2004. "Informed Consent in Acute Myocardial Infarction Research." *Journal of Medicine and Philosophy* 29 (4): 417–34. https://doi.org/10.1080/03605310490503533.

Geissler, P. Wenzel. 2013. "Public Secrets in Public Health: Knowing Not to Know While Making Scientific Knowledge." *American Ethnologist* 40 (1): 13–34. https://doi.org/10.1111/amet.12002.

Geissler, P. Wenzel, and Sassy Molyneux, eds. 2011. *Evidence, Ethos and Experiment: The Anthropology and History of Medical Research in Africa*. New York: Berghahn Books.

Ghaffar, Abdul, K. Srinath Reddy, and Monica Singhi. 2004. "Burden of Non-Communicable Diseases in South Asia." *BMJ* 328 (7443): 807–10. https://doi.org/10.1136/bmj.328.7443.807.

Gibbons, Michael, Camille Limoges, Helga Nowotny, Simon Schwartzman, Peter Scott, and Martin Trow. 1994. *The New Production of Knowledge: The Dynamics of Science and Research in Contemporary Societies*. London: Sage.

Gikonyo, Caroline, Philip Bejon, Vicki M. Marsh, and Sassy Molyneux. 2008. "Taking Social Relationships Seriously: Lessons Learned from the Informed Consent Practices of a Vaccine Trial on the Kenyan Coast." *Social Science and Medicine* 67: 708–20. https://doi.org/10.1016/j.socscimed.2008.02.003.

Glickman, Seth W., John G. McHutchison, Eric D. Peterson, Charles B. Cairns, Robert A. Harrington, Robert M. Califf, and Kevin A. Schulman. 2009. "Ethical and Scientific Implications of the Globalization of Clinical Research." *New England Journal of Medicine* 360 (8): 816–23. https://doi.org/10.1056/NEJMsb0803929.

Goodwin, L. G., L. G. Jayewardene, and O. D. Standen. 1958. "Clinical Trials with Bephenium Hydroxynaphthoate against Hookworm in Ceylon." *British Medical Journal* 2 (5112): 1572–76. https://doi.org/10.1136/bmj.2.5112.1572.

Goonatilake, Susantha. 1998. *Toward a Global Science: Mining Civilizational Knowledge.* Bloomington: Indiana University Press.

Graboyes, Melissa. 2014. "Introduction: Incorporating Medical Research into the History of Medicine in East Africa." *International Journal of African Historical Studies* 47 (3): 379–98. http://www.jstor.org/stable/24393435.

———. 2015. *The Experiment Must Continue: Medical Research and Ethics in East Africa, 1940–2014.* Columbus: Ohio University Press.

Gunawardene, N. 1999. "Sri Lanka's Double Burden Kills Rich and Poor Alike." *Health for the Millions* 25 (4): 27. http://www.popline.org/node/523623.

Gunnell, D., and M. Eddleston. 2003. "Suicide by Intentional Ingestion of Pesticides: A Continuing Tragedy in Developing Countries." *International Journal of Epidemiology* 32 (6): 902–9. https://doi.org/10.1093/ije/dyg307.

Gunnell, D., M. Eddleston, M. Phillips, and F. Konradsen. 2007. "The Global Distribution of Fatal Pesticide Self-Poisoning: Systematic Review." *BMC Public Health* 7: 357. https://doi.org/10.1186/1471-2458-7-357.

Gunnell, D., R. Fernando, M. Hewagama, W. D. D. Priyangika, F. Konradsen, and M. Eddleston. 2007. "The Impact of Pesticide Regulations on Suicide in Sri Lanka." *International Journal of Epidemiology* 36: 1235–42. https://doi.org/10.1093/ije/dym164.

Haines, Andy, Shyama Kuruvilla, and Matthias Borchert. 2004. "Bridging the Implementation Gap between Knowledge and Action for Health." *Bulletin of the World Health Organization* 82 (10): 724–31. https://doi.org/10.1590/S0042-96862004001000005.

Harding, Sandra. 2008. *Sciences from Below: Feminisms, Postcolonialities, and Modernities.* Durham, NC: Duke University Press.

Harrison, Mark. 2010. *Medicine in an Age of Commerce and Empire: Britain and Its Tropical Colonies 1660–1830.* Oxford: Oxford University Press.

Heckler, S., and A. Russell. 2008. "Confronting Collaboration: Dilemmas in an Ethnographic Study of Health Policy Makers." *Anthropology in Action* 15 (1): 14–21. https://doi.org/10.3167/aia.2008.150104.

Hedgecoe, A. M. 2004. "Critical Bioethics: Beyond the Social Science Critique of Applied Ethics." *Bioethics* 18 (2): 120–43. https://doi.org/10.1111/j.1467-8519.2004.00385.x.

Helgesson, C. F. 2010. "From Dirty Data to Credible Scientific Evidence: Some Practices Used to Clean Data in Large Randomised Clinical Trials." In *Medical Proofs/ Social Experiments: Clinical Trials in Context,* edited by C. Will and T. Moreira, 49–63. Aldershot, United Kingdom: Ashgate.

Hess, David. 2001. "Ethnography and the Development of Science and Technology Studies." In *Handbook of Ethnography*, edited by Paul Atkinson, Amanda Coffey, Sarah Delamont, Paul Lofland, and Lyn Lofland, 234–45. London: Sage.

Hewa, Soma. 1995. *Colonialism, Tropical Disease, and Imperial Medicine: Rockefeller Philanthropy in Sri Lanka*. Lanham, NY: University Press of America.

———. 2012. "The Hookworm Epidemic on the Plantations in Colonial Sri Lanka." *Medical History* 38 (1): 73–90. https://doi.org/10.1017/S0025727300056052.

Hewlett, Christopher. 2017. "Community Capacity Building: Transforming Amerindian Sociality in Peruvian Amazonia." *Cambridge Anthropology* 35 (1): 114–30.

Hill, Austin Bradford. 1990. "Memories of the British Streptomycin Trial in Tuberculosis." *Controlled Clinical Trials* 11 (2): 77–79. https://doi.org/10.1016/0197-2456 (90)90001-I.

Holden, Kerry and David Demeritt. 2008. "Democratising Science? The Politics of Promoting Biomedicine in Singapore's Developmental State." *Environment and Planning D: Society and Space* 26 (1): 68–86. https://doi.org/10.1068/d461t.

Holmes, Douglas R., and George E. Marcus. 2005. "Refunctioning Ethnography: The Challenge of an Anthropology of the Contemporary." In *The Sage Handbook of Qualitative Research*, edited by N. Denzin and Y. Lincoln, 1099–111. Thousand Oaks, CA: Sage.

———. 2008a. "Collaboration Today and the Re-Imagination of the Classic Scene of Fieldwork Encounter." *Collaborative Anthropologies* 1 (1): 81–101. https://doi.org/10 .1353/cla.0.0003.

———. 2009b. "Para-Ethnography." In *The Sage Encyclopedia of Qualitative Research*, edited by Lisa M. Given, 595–97. London: Sage.

Hyder, Adnan A., and Salman A. Wali. 2006. "Informed Consent and Collaborative Research: Perspectives from the Developing World." *Developing World Bioethics* 6 (1): 33–40.

Iivonen, M., and D. H. Sonnenwald. 2000. "The Use of Technology in International Collaboration: Two Case Studies." *Proceedings of the ASIS Annual Meeting* 37: 78–92. http://eric.ed.gov/?id=EJ618404.

Ingold, Timothy. 2001. "From the Transmission of Representations to the Education of Attention." In *The Debated Mind: Evolutionary Psychology versus Ethnography*, edited by H. Whitehouse, 113–53. Oxford: Berghahn Books.

Institute for Research and Development. 2014. "About." http://www.ird.lk/about-ird/.

Jansen, L. A., and S. Wall. 2009. "Paternalism and Fairness in Clinical Research." *Bioethics* 23 (3): 172–82. https://doi.org/10.1111/j.1467-8519.2008.00651.x.

Jasanoff, Sheila. 2005. *Designs on Nature: Science and Democracy in Europe and the United States*. Princeton, NJ: Princeton University Press.

———. 2014. "Biotechnology and Empire: The Global Power of Seeds and Science." In *The Global Politics of Science and Technology*, Vol. 1, edited by M. Mayer, M. Carpes, and R. Knoblich, 201–25. Berlin: Springer. http://link.springer.com/chapter/10.1007 /978-3-642-55007-2_10.

Jayasekara, Rasika S., and Tim Schultz. 2007. "Health Status, Trends, and Issues in Sri Lanka." *Nursing and Health Sciences* 9 (3): 228–33. https://doi.org/10.1111/j.1442-2018 .2007.00328.x.

Jayasinghe, Saroj. 2002. "Context of the Health Care System." In *Health Sector in Sri Lanka: Current Status and Changes*, 1–11. Colombo, Sri Lanka: Health Development and Research Programme.

Jeffery, Patricia., and Roger. Jeffery. 1996. *Don't Marry Me to a Plowman!: Women's Everyday Lives in Rural North India*. Boulder, CO: Westview Press.

Johnson, R., and A. Khalid, eds. 2012. *Public Health in the British Empire: Intermediaries, Subordinates, and the Practice of Public Health, 1850–1960*. London: Routledge.

Jones, Margaret. 2000. "The Ceylon Malaria Epidemic of 1934–35: A Case Study in Colonial Medicine." *Social History of Medicine* 13 (1): 87–110. https://doi.org/10.1093/shm/13.1.87.

Jonsen, Albert. R. 1998. *The Birth of Bioethics*. New York: Oxford University Press.

Kamat, Vinay R. 2014. "Fast, Cheap, and out of Control? Speculations and Ethical Concerns in the Conduct of Outsourced Clinical Trials in India." *Social Science and Medicine* 104 (March): 48–55. https://doi.org/10.1016/j.socscimed.2013.12.008.

Kamuya, Dorcas M., Vicki M. Marsh, Patricia Njuguna, Patrick Munywoki, Michael Parker, and Sassy Molyneux. 2014. "'When They See Us, It's Like They Have Seen the Benefits!': Experiences of Study Benefits Negotiations in Community-Based Studies on the Kenyan Coast." *BMC Medical Ethics* 15 (1): 90. https://doi.org/10.1186/1472-6939-15-90.

Kamuya, Dorcas M., Sally J. Theobald, Patrick K. Munywoki, Dorothy Koech, P. Wenzel Geissler, and Sassy C Molyneux. 2013. "Evolving Friendships and Shifting Ethical Dilemmas: Fieldworkers' Experiences in a Short Term Community Based Study in Kenya." *Developing World Bioethics* 13 (1): 1–9. https://doi.org/10.1111/dewb.12009.

Kapferer, B. 1983. *A Celebration of Demons: Exorcism and the Aesthetics of Healing in Sri Lanka*. Bloomington: Indiana Press.

Karunanayake, Panduka. 2012. "Global Clinical Trials: Effective Participant Protection Must Be Ensured." *The Island*, September 8. http://www.island.lk/index.php?page_cat=article-details&page=article-details&code_title=60904.

Kearney, R. N., and B. D. Miller. 1985. "The Spiral of Suicide and Social Change in Sri Lanka." *Journal of Asian Studies* 45 (1): 81–101. https://doi.org/10.2307/2056825.

Kelly, Ann H. 2015. "The Territory of Medical Research: Experimentation in Africa's Smallest State." In *Para-States and Medical Science: Making African Global Health*, edited by Paul Wenzel Geissler, 303–33. Durham, NC: Duke University Press.

Kelly, A. & Beisel, U. 2011. *BioSocieties* 6 (1): 71–87. https://doi.org/10.1057/biosoc.2010.42.

Kilpatrick, D. G. 2004. "The Ethics of Disaster Research: A Special Section." *Journal of Traumatic Stress* 17 (5): 361–62. https://doi.org/10.1023/B:JOTS.0000048961.75301.74.

Kingori, Patricia. 2013. "Experiencing Everyday Ethics in Context: Frontline Data Collectors Perspectives and Practices of Bioethics." *Social Science and Medicine* 98: 361–70. https://doi.org/10.1016/j.socscimed.2013.10.013.

——. 2015. "The 'Empty Choice': A Sociological Examination of Choosing Medical Research Participation in Resource-Limited Sub-Saharan Africa." *Current Sociology* 63 (5): 763–78. https://doi.org/10.1177/0011392115590093.

Kingori, Patricia, and René Gerrets. 2016. "Morals, Morale and Motivations in Data Fabrication: Medical Research Fieldworkers Views and Practices in Two Sub-Saharan

African Contexts." *Social Science and Medicine* 166 (October): 150–59. https://doi.org /10.1016/j.socscimed.2016.08.019.

Kingori, Patricia, and Salla Sariola. 2015. "Museum of Failed HIV Research." *Anthropology and Medicine* 22 (3): 213–16. https://doi.org/10.1080/13648470.2015.1079302.

Kipnis, Kenneth. 2001. "Vulnerability in Research Subjects: A Bioethical Taxonomy." In *Ethical and Policy Issues in Research Involving Human Subjects*, Vol. 2: *Commissioned Papers and Staff Analysis*, G1–G13. Bethesda, MD: National Bioethics Advisory Commission. https://repository.library.georgetown.edu/bitstream/handle/10822/559361/nbac _human_part_vol2.pdf.

Kleinman, A. 1995. *Writing at the Margin: Discourse Between Anthropology and Medicine.* Berkeley: University of California Press.

——. 2006. "Ethics and Experience: An Anthropological Approach to Health Equity." In *Public Health, Ethics, and Equity*, edited by Sudhir Anand, Fabienne Peter, and Amartya Sen, 269–82. Oxford: Oxford University Press.

Kleinman, A., and E. Fitz-Henry. 2007. "The Experiential Basis of Subjectivity: How Individuals Change in the Context of Societal Transformation." In *Subjectivity: Ethnographic Investigations*, edited by João G. Biehl, B. Good, and Arthur Kleinman, 52–65. Berkeley: University of California Press.

Knorr-Cetina, K. 1999. *Epistemic Cultures: How the Sciences Make Knowledge.* Mass: Harvard University Press.

Komrad, M. S. 1983. "A Defence of Medical Paternalism: Maximising Patients' Autonomy." *Journal of Medical Ethics* 9 (1): 38–44. https://doi.org/10.1136/jme.9.1.38.

Konrad, Monica, ed. 2012. *Collaborators Collaborating: Counterparts in Anthropological Knowledge and International Research Relations.* New York: Berghahn Books.

Konradsen, F., W. van der Hoek, and P. Peiris. 2006. "Reaching for the Bottle of Pesticide—A Cry for Help. Self-Inflicted Poisonings in Sri Lanka." *Social Science and Medicine* 62 (7): 1710–19. https://doi.org/10.1016/j.socscimed.2005.08.020.

Kristeva, Julia. 1982. *Powers of Horror: An Essay on Abjection.* Translated by Leon S. Roudiez. New York: Colombia University Press.

LaHatte, Kristin. 2017. Professionalizing Persons and Foretelling Futures: Capacity Building in Post-Earthquake Haiti. *Cambridge Anthropology* 35 (1): 17–30.

Laidlaw, J. 2014. *The Subject of Virtue: An Anthropology of Ethics and Freedom.* Cambridge: Cambridge University Press.

Lairumbi, Geoffrey Mbaabu, Sassy Molyneux, Robert W. Snow, Kevin Marsh, Norbert Peshu, and Mike English. 2008. "Promoting the Social Value of Research in Kenya: Examining the Practical Aspects of Collaborative Partnerships Using an Ethical Framework." *Social Science and Medicine* 67 (5): 734–47. https://doi.org/10.1016/j .socscimed.2008.02.016.

Lairumbi, Geoffrey Mbaabu, M. Parker, Raymond Fitzpatrick, and Michael C. English. 2012. "Forms of Benefit Sharing in Global Health Research Undertaken in Resource Poor Settings: A Qualitative Study of Stakeholders' Views in Kenya." *Philosophy, Ethics, and Humanities in Medicine* 7 (7): 1–8. http://www.peh-med.com/content/7/1/7.

Lakoff, Andrew. 2010. "Two Regimes of Global Health." *Humanity: An International Journal of Human Rights, Humanitarianism, and Development* 1 (1): 59–79. https://doi .org/10.1353/hum.2010.0001.

Lall, Sanjaya. 1977. "The Political Economy of Controlling Transnationals: The Pharmaceutical Industry in Sri Lanka (1972–1976)." *World Development* 5 (8): 677–97. https://doi.org/10.1016/0305-750X(77)90085-7.

Laloe, V., and M. Ganesan. 2002. "Self-Immolation a Common Suicidal Behaviour in Eastern Sri Lanka." *Burns* 28: 475–80. https://doi.org/10.1016/S0305-4179(02)00047-5.

Lamb, S. 1997. "The Making and Unmaking of Persons: Notes on Aging and Gender in North India." *Ethos* 25 (3): 279–302. https://doi.org/10.1525/eth.1997.25.3.279.

Lambek, Michael, ed. 2010. *Ordinary Ethics: Anthropology, Language, and Action.* New York: Fordham University Press.

———. 2013. "The Continuous and Discontinuous Person: Two Dimensions of Ethical Life." *Journal of the Royal Anthropological Institute* 19 (4): 837–58. https://doi.org/10.1111/1467-9655.12073.

Lang, Trudie, and Sisira Siribaddana. 2012. "Clinical Trials Have Gone Global: Is This a Good Thing?" *PLoS Medicine* 9 (6): e1001228. https://doi.org/10.1371/journal.pmed.1001228.

Latour, Bruno. 1982. "Give Me a Laboratory and I Will Raise the World." In *Science Observed*, edited by K. Knorr and M. Mulkay, 141–70. London: Sage.

———. 1987. *Science in Action: How to Follow Scientists and Engineers through Society.* Milton Keynes, United Kingdom: Open University Press.

———. 1993. *We Have Never Been Modern.* Cambridge MA: Harvard University Press.

———. 2005. *Reassembling the Social: An Introduction to Actor-Network-Theory.* Oxford: Oxford University Press.

Lave, Jean, and Etienne Wenger. 1991. *Situated Learning: Legitimate Peripheral Participation.* Cambridge: Cambridge University Press.

Leach, Melissa, Ian Scoones, and Brian Wynne, 2005. *Science and Citizens: Globalization and the Challenge of Engagement.* London: Zed Books.

Le Marcis, F. 2015. "Life Promises and 'Failed' Family Ties: Expectations and Disappointment within a Clinical Trial (Ivory Coast)." *Anthropology and Medicine* 22 (3): 295–308. https://doi.org/10.1080/13648470.2015.1081671.

Löwy, Ilana. 2011. "The Best Possible Intentions Testing Prophylactic Approaches on Humans in Developing Countries." *American Journal of Public Health* 103 (2): 226–37. https://doi.org/10.2105/AJPH.2012.300901.

Macklin, Ruth. 2004. *Double Standards in Medical Research in Developing Countries.* Cambridge: Cambridge University Press.

Malkki, Liisa H. 1996. "Speechless Emissaries: Refugees, Humanitarianism, and Dehistoricization." *Cultural Anthropology* 11 (3): 377–404. https://doi.org/10.1525/can.1996.11.3.02a00050.

Manton, John. 2011. "Testing a New Drug for Leprosy: Clofazimine and Its Precursors in Ireland and Nigeria, 1944–1966." In *Evidence, Ethos and Experiment: The Anthropology and History of Medical Research in Africa*, edited by P. Wenzel Geissler and Sassy Molyneux, 125–58. New York: Berghahn Books.

Manuel, Celie, David J. Gunnell, Wim van der Hoek, Andrew Dawson, Ishika K. Wijeratne, and Flemming Konradsen. 2008. "Self-Poisoning in Rural Sri Lanka: Small-Area Variations in Incidence." *BMC Public Health* 8 (1): 26. https://doi.org/10.1186/1471-2458-8-26.

Marcus, George E., ed. 2000. *Para-Sites: A Casebook against Cynical Reason*. Chicago: University of Chicago Press.

———. 2005. "The Passion of Anthropology in the U.S., Circa 2004." *Anthropological Quarterly* 78 (3): 673–95. https://doi.org/10.1353/anq.2005.0036.

———. 2013. "Experimental Forms for the Expression of Norms in the Ethnography of the Contemporary." *HAU: Journal of Ethnographic Theory* 3 (2): 197–217. https://doi.org/10.14318/hau3.2.011.

Marecek, Jeanne. 1998. "Culture, Gender, and Suicidal Behavior in Sri Lanka." *Suicide and Life-Threatening Behavior* 28 (1): 69–82. https://doi.org/10.1111/j.1943-278X.1998.tb00627.x.

———. 2000. "Resisting and Remaking Gender Imperatives: Women's Suicide as Gendered Protest in Sri Lanka." *International Journal of Psychology* 35 (3–4): 63–92.

———. 2006. "Young Women's Suicides In Sri Lanka: Cultural, Ecological and Psychological Factors." *Asian Journal of Counselling* 13 (1): 63–92.

Marks, Harry M. 1997. *The Progress of Experiment: Science and Therapeutic Reform in the United States, 1900–1990*. Cambridge: Cambridge University Press.

Marriott, McKim. 1976. "Hindu Transactions: Diversity without Dualism." In *Transaction and Meaning: Directions in the Anthropology of Exchange and Symbolic Behavior*, edited by B. Kapferer, 109–42. Philadelphia: Institute for the Study of Human Issues.

Marsh, Vicki M., Dorcas Kamuya, Yvonne Rowa, Caroline Gikonyo, and Sassy Molyneux. 2008. "Beginning Community Engagement at a Busy Biomedical Research Programme: Experiences from the KEMRI CGMRC-Wellcome Trust Research Programme, Kilifi, Kenya." *Social Science and Medicine* 67: 721–33. https://doi.org/10.1016/j.socscimed.2008.02.007.

Marshall, Patricia A. 1992. "Anthropology and Bioethics." *Medical Anthropology Quarterly* 6 (1): 49–73. https://doi.org/10.1525/maq.1992.6.1.02a00040.

Martin, Brian. 2005. "Agricultural Antibiotics: Features of a Controversy." In *Controversies in Science and Technology: From Maize to Menopause*, edited by Abby J. Kinchy and Jo Handelsman, 37–51. Madison: University of Wisconsin Press.

———. 2008. "The Globalisation of Scientific Controversy." *Globalization* 7 (1):no pagination. http://globalization.icaap.org/content/v7.1/Martin.html.

Martin, Brian, and E. Richards. 1995. "Scientific Knowledge, Controversy, and Public Decision-Making." In *Handbook of Science and Technology Studies*, edited by Sheila Jasanoff, Gerald E. Markle, James C. Petersen, and Trevor Pinch, 506–26. Thousand Oaks, CA: Sage.

Mauss, Marcel. (1938) 1985. "The Category of the Human Mind: The Notion of the Person; The Notion of the Self." In *The Category of the Person: Anthropology, Philosophy, History*, edited by Michael Carrithers, Steven Collins, and Steven Lukes, 1–25. Cambridge: Cambridge University Press.

Mayhew, Susannah H., Jane Doherty, Siriwan Pitayarangsarit, B. Maina-Ahlberg, E. Nordberg, G. Tomson, E. Harris, et al. 2008. "Developing Health Systems Research Capacities through North-South Partnership: An Evaluation of Collaboration with South Africa and Thailand." *Health Research Policy and Systems* 6 (8): 1–12. https://doi.org/10.1186/1478-4505-6-8.

Mazur, Allan. 1975. "Opposition to Technological Innovation." *Minerva* 13 (1): 58–81. https://doi.org/10.1007/BF01096242.

———. 1981. "Media Coverage and Public Opinion on Scientific Controversies." *Journal of Communication* 31 (2): 106–15. https://doi.org/10.1111/j.1460-2466.1981.tb01234.x.

McGoey, Linsey. 2012. "The Logic of Strategic Ignorance." *British Journal of Sociology* 63: 533–76. https://doi.org/10.1111/j.1468-4446.2012.01424.x.

———. 2014. "The Philanthropic State: Market–State Hybrids in the Philanthrocapitalist Turn." *Third World Quarterly* 35 (1): 109–25. http://www.tandfonline.com/doi/abs/10.1080/01436597.2014.868989.

McGoey, Linsey, Julian Reiss, and Ayo Wahlberg. 2011. "Editors' Intro: The Global Health Complex." *BioSocieties* 6 (1): 106–18. https://doi.org/10.1057/biosoc.2010.44.

McIntosh, S., E. Sierra, A. Dozier, S. Diaz, Z. Qionones, A. Primack, G. Chadwick, and D. Ossip-Klein. 2008. "Ethical Review Issues in Collaborative Research between US and Low–Middle Income Country Partners: A Case Example." *Bioethics* 22 (8): 414–22. https://doi.org/10.1111/j.1467-8519.2008.00662.x.

Medawar, P. B. 1967. *The Art of the Soluble.* Oxford: Oxford University Press. http://philpapers.org/rec/MEDPRI.

Medical Research Council (MRC). 1948. "Streptomycin Treatment of Pulmonary Tuberculosis: A Medical Research Council Investigation." *British Medical Journal* 2 (4582): 769–82. http://www.jstor.org/stable/25365309.

Melin, Göran. 2000. "Pragmatism and Self-Organization." *Research Policy* 29 (1): 31–40. https://doi.org/10.1016/S0048-7333(99)00031-1.

Mendis, Shirmila, and Saroj Jayasinghe. 2002. "Labels, Packages and Leaflets in Drugs and Devices: The Language Matters a Lot." *Ceylon Medical Journal* 47 (3): 100. https://dx.doi.org/10.4038/cmj.v47i3.3441.

Merton, Robert K. (1942) 1973. "The Normative Structure of Science." In *The Sociology of Science: Theoretical and Empirical Investigations*, 267–78. Chicago: University of Chicago Press.

Miller, F. G., and A. Wertheimer. 2007. "Facing up to Paternalism in Research Ethics." *Hastings Center Report* 37 (3): 24–34. https://doi.org/10.1353/hcr.2007.0044.

Mines, M. 1988. "Conceptualizing the Person: Hierarchical Society and Individual Autonomy in India." *American Anthropologist* 90 (3): 568–79. https://doi.org/10.1525/aa.1988.90.3.02a00030.

Mohanty, B. B. 2005. "'We Are Like the Living Dead': Farmer Suicides in Maharashtra, Western India." *Journal of Peasant Studies* 32 (2): 243–76. https://doi.org/10.1080/03066150500094485.

Molyneux, C. S., N. Peshu, and K. Marsh. 2005a. "Trust and Informed Consent: Insights from Community Members on the Kenyan Coast." *Social Science and Medicine* 61: 1463–73. https://doi.org/10.1016/j.socscimed.2004.11.073.

Molyneux, C. S., D. R. Wassenaar, N. Peshu, and K. Marsh. 2005b. "'Even If They Ask You to Stand by a Tree All Day, You Will Have to Do It (Laughter)!': Community Voices on the Notion and Practice of Informed Consent for Biomedical Research in Developing Countries." *Social Science and Medicine* 61: 443–54. https://doi.org/10.1016/j.socscimed.2004.12.003.

Molyneux, C. S., Dorcas Kamuya, Philister Adhiambo Madiega, Tracey Chantler, Vibian Angwenyi, and P. Wenzel Geissler. 2013. "Field Workers at the Interface." *Developing World Bioethics* 13 (1): ii–iv. https://doi.org/10.1111/dewb.12027.

Montgomery, Catherine M. 2015. "'HIV Has a Woman's Face': Vaginal Microbicides and a Case of Ambiguous Failure." *Anthropology and Medicine* 22 (3): 250–62. https://doi.org/10.1080/13648470.2015.1077200.

Montgomery, Catherine M., and Robert Pool. 2017. "From 'Trial Community' to 'Experimental Publics': How Clinical Research Shapes Public Participation." *Critical Public Health* 27 (1): 50–62. https://doi.org/10.1080/09581596.2016.1212161.

Moreira, T., and C. Will, eds. 2010. *Medical Proofs, Social Experiments: Clinical Trials in Shifting Contexts.* Aldershot, United Kingdom: Ashgate.

Mosse, D. 2005. *Cultivating Development: An Ethnography of Aid Policy and Practice.* London: Pluto.

Mueller, M. R. 1997. "2. Science versus Care: Physicians, Nurses, and the Dilemma of Clinical Research." *Sociology of Health and Illness* 19: 57–78. https://doi.org/10.1111/1467-9566.00086.

Muller, Jessica H. 1994. "Anthropology, Bioethics, and Medicine: A Provocative Trilogy." *Medical Anthropology Quarterly* 8 (4): 448–67. http://www.jstor.org/stable/649090.

Myser, Catherine. 2007. "White Normativity in United States Bioethics: A Call and Method for More Pluralist and Democratic Standards and Policies." In *The Ethics of Bioethics: Mapping the Moral Landscape*, edited by L. A. Eckenwiler and F. G. Cohn, 241–59. Baltimore: Johns Hopkins University Press.

———. 2011. "Introduction: First Steps toward a Comparative Anthropology and Sociology of Globalizing Bioethics—Reflections on Cultural Meanings and Social Functions of Bioethics." In *Bioethics around the Globe*, edited by Catherine Myser, xix–xxxiv. Oxford: Oxford University Press.

National Commission for the Protection of Human Subjects of Biomedical and Behavioral Research. 1978. *The Belmont Report: Ethical Principles and Guidelines for the Protection of Human Subjects of Research.* Washington, DC: Department of Health, Education, and Welfare. https://videocast.nih.gov/pdf/ohrp_belmont_report.pdf.

National Science and Technology Commission (NASTEC). 2003. *New Genetics and Assisted Reproductive Technologies in Sri Lanka: A Draft National Policy on Biomedical Ethics.* Colombo, Sri Lanka: National Science and Technology Commission.

Nelkin, Dorothy. 1984. *Controversy: Politics of Technical Decisions.* London: Sage.

Nguyen, Vinh-Kim. 2005. "Antiretroviral Globalism, Biopolitics, and Therapeutic Citizenship." In *Global Assemblages: Technology, Politics, and Ethics as Anthropological Problems*, 124–44. London: Blackwell.

Njue, M., F. Kombe, S. Mwalukore, S. Molyneux, and Vicki M. Marsh. 2014. "What Are Fair Study Benefits in International Health Research? Consulting Community Members in Kenya." *PloS One* 9 (12): e113112. https://doi.org/10.1371/journal.pone.0113112.

Nowotny, Helga, and Helmut Hirsch. 1980. "The Consequences of Dissent: Sociological Reflections on the Controversy of the Low Dose Effects." *Research Policy* 9 (3): 278–94. https://doi.org/10.1016/0048-7333(80)90004-9.

Nowotny, Helga, P. Scott, and M. Gibbons. 2001. *Re-Thinking Science: Knowledge and the Public in an Age of Uncertainty.* Oxford: Polity Press.

Nuffield Council on Bioethics. 2002. "The Ethics of Research Related to Health Care in Developing Countries." London: Nuffield Council on Bioethics.

Ong, A., and S. J. Collier. 2005. *Global Assemblages: Technology, Politics, and Ethics as Anthropological Problems.* Oxford: Blackwell.

Parker, Michael, and Patricia Kingori. 2016. "Good and Bad Research Collaborations: Researchers' Views on Science and Ethics in Global Health Research." Edited by Anny Fortin. *PLOS One* 11 (10): e0163579. https://doi.org/10.1371/journal.pone.0163579.

Patel, Vikram, Chinthanie Ramasundarahettige, Lakshmi Vijayakumar, J. S. Thakur, Vendhan Gajalakshmi, Gopalkrishna Gururaj, Wilson Suraweera, and Prabhat Jha. 2012. "Suicide Mortality in India: A Nationally Representative Survey." *Lancet* 379 (9834): 2343–51. https://doi.org/10.1016/S0140-6736(12)60606-0.

Pearson, Melissa, Anthony B. Zwi, Nicholas A. Buckley, Gamini Manuweera, Ravindra Fernando, Andrew H. Dawson, and Duncan McDuie-Ra. 2015. "Policymaking 'Under the Radar': A Case Study of Pesticide Regulation to Prevent Intentional Poisoning in Sri Lanka." *Health Policy and Planning* 30 (1): 56–67. https://doi.org/10.1093/heapol/czt096.

Petryna, Adriana. 2005. "Ethical Variability: Drug Development and Globalizing Clinical Trials." *American Ethnologist* 32 (2): 183–97. http://www.jstor.org/stable/3805277.

——. 2007a. "Clinical Trials Offshored: On Private Sector Science and Public Health." *BioSocieties* 2: 21–40. https://doi.org/10.1017/S1745855207005030.

——. 2007b. "Experimentality: On the Global Mobility and Regulation of Human Subjects Research." *PoLAR: Political and Legal Anthropology Review* 30 (2): 288–304. https://doi.org/10.1525/pol.2007.30.2.288.

——. 2009. *When Experiments Travel: Clinical Trials and the Global Search for Human Subjects.* Princeton, NJ: Princeton University Press.

Petty, J. L., and C. A. Heimer. 2011. "Extending the Rails: How Research Reshapes Clinics." *Social Studies of Science* 41 (3): 337–60. https://doi.org/10.1177/0306312710396402.

Pfeiffer, James. 2003. "International NGOs and Primary Health Care in Mozambique: The Need for a New Model of Collaboration." *Social Science and Medicine* 56 (4): 725–38. https://doi.org/10.1016/S0277-9536(02)00068-0.

Phillips, J. 2006. "Agencement/Assemblage." *Theory, Culture and Society* 23 (2–3): 108–9. https://doi.org/10.1177/026327640602300219.

Phillips, Rodney E., R. David Theakston, David A. Warrell, Yamuna Galigedara, D. T. D. J. Abeysekera, P. Dissanayaka, Ronald A. Hutton, and Dennis J. Aloysius. 1988. "Paralysis, Rhabdomyolysis and Haemolysis Caused by Bites of Russell's Viper (*Vipera russelli pulchella*) in Sri Lanka: Failure of Indian (Haffkine) Antivenom." *QJM* 68 (257): 691–715. https://doi.org/10.1093/oxfordjournals.qjmed.a068236.

Pieris, Kamalika. 2001. *The Medical Profession in Sri Lanka 1843–1980.* Colombo, Sri Lanka: Visidunu Prakashakayo.

Polanyi, M. 1958. *Personal Knowledge: Towards a Post-Critical Philosophy.* London: Routledge and Kegan Paul.

Pollock, Anne. 2014. "Places of Pharmaceutical Knowledge-Making: Global Health, Postcolonial Science, and Hope in South African Drug Discovery." *Social Studies of Science* 44 (6): 848–73. https://doi.org/10.1177/0306312714543285.

Powdermaker, H. 1966. *Stranger and Friend: The Way of an Anthropologist.* New York: W. W. Norton.

Prainsack, B., M. N. Svendsen, L. Koch, and K. Ehrich. 2010. "How Do We Collaborate? Social Science Researchers' Experience of Multidisciplinarity in Biomedical Settings." *BioSocieties* 5 (2): 278–86. https://doi.org/10.1057/biosoc.2010.7.

Prasad, Amit. 2006. "Beyond Modern versus Alternative Science Debate: Analysis of Magnetic Resonance Imaging Research." *Economic and Political Weekly* 41 (3): 219–27.

———. 2009. "Capitalizing Disease." *Theory, Culture and Society* 26 (5): 1–29. https://doi.org/10.1177/0263276409106347.

———. 2014. *Imperial Technoscience: Transnational Histories of MRI in the United States, Britain, and India.* Cambridge, MA: MIT Press.

Rabinow, Paul, George E. Marcus, James D. Faubion, and Tobias Rees. 2008. *Designs for an Anthropology of the Contemporary.* Durham, NC: Duke University Press.

Rahula, Walpola. 1978. *Zen and the Taming of the Bull: Towards the Definition of Buddhist Thought: Essays.* Surrey, United Kingdom: Gordon Fraser.

Raj, Kapil. 2013. "Beyond Postcolonialism . . . and Postpositivism: Circulation and the Global History of Science." *Isis* 104 (2): 337–47. https://doi.org/10.1086/670951.

Rannan-Eliya, Ravi P., and Lankani Sikurajapathy. 2009. "Sri Lanka: 'Good Practice' in Expanding Health Care Coverage." Washington, DC: International Bank for Reconstruction and Development/World Bank. http://www.ihp.lk/publications/docs/RSS0903.pdf.

Ratnayeke, L. 1996. "Suicide and Crisis Intervention in Rural Communities in Sri Lanka." *Crisis* 17 (4): 149–51, 154. https://doi.org/10.1027/0227-5910.17.4.149.

Reader, S. 2010. "Agency, Patiency, and Personhood." In *A Companion to the Philosophy of Action*, edited by Timothy O'Connor and Constantine Sandis, 200–8. Oxford: Wiley-Blackwell. https://doi.org/10.1002/9781444323528.ch26.

Reed, Adam. 2011. "Inspiring Strathern." In *Recasting Anthropological Knowledge: Inspiration and Social Science*, edited by Jeanette Edwards and Maja Petrovic-Steger, 165–83. Cambridge: Cambridge University Press.

Reilley, B., R. Abeyasinghe, and M. Vincent Pakianathar. 2002. "Barriers to Prompt and Effective Treatment of Malaria in Northern Sri Lanka." *Tropical Medicine and International Health* 7 (9): 744–49. https://doi.org/10.1046/j.1365-3156.2002.00919.x.

Rose, Nikolas. 2007. *The Politics of Life Itself: Biomedicine, Power, and Subjectivity in the Twenty-First Century.* Princeton, NJ: Princeton University Press.

Rosemann, A., and N. Chaisinthop. 2015. "The Pluralization of the International: Resistance and Alter-Standardization in Regenerative Stem Cell Medicine." *Social Studies of Science* 46 (1): 112–39. https://doi.org/10.1177/0306312715619783.

Royal Society. 2017. "The Role of International Collaboration and Mobility in Research." *Opinion Leader*, May 4, https://royalsociety.org/~/media/policy/projects/international-mobility/national-academies-opinion-leader-survey.pdf.

Russell, Steven. 2005. "Treatment-Seeking Behaviour in Urban Sri Lanka: Trusting the State, Trusting Private Providers." *Social Science and Medicine* 61 (7): 1396–1407. https://doi.org/10.1016/j.socscimed.2004.11.077.

Sambakunsi, Rodrick, Moses Kumwenda, Augustine Choko, Elizabeth L Corbett, and Nicola Ann Desmond. 2015. "'Whose Failure Counts?' A Critical Reflection on Definitions of Failure for Community Health Volunteers Providing HIV Self-Testing in a Community-Based HIV/TB Intervention Study in Urban Malawi." *Anthropology and Medicine* 22 (3): 234–49. https://doi.org/10.1080/13648470.2015.1077202.

Sariola, Salla, Roger Jeffery, Amar Jesani, and Gerard Porter. 2018. "How Civil Society Organisations Changed the Regulation of Clinical Trials in India." *Science as Culture*, published online August 13, 2018. DOI: 10.1080/09505431.2018.1493449.

Sariola, Salla, Deapica Ravindran, Anand Kumar, and Roger Jeffery. 2015. "Big-Pharmaceuticalisation: Clinical Trials and Contract Research Organisations in India." *Social Science and Medicine* 131 (April): 239–46. https://doi.org/10.1016/j.socscimed.2014.11.052.

Schlecker, Markus, and Eric Hirsch. 2001. "Incomplete Knowledge: Ethnography and the Crisis of Context in Studies of Media, Science and Technology." *History of the Human Sciences* 14 (1): 69–87. https://doi.org/10.1177/095269510101400104.

Simon, David, Duncan McGregor, Kwasi Nsiah-Gyabaah, and Donald Thompson. 2003. "Poverty Elimination, North-South Research Collaboration, and the Politics of Participatory Development." *Development in Practice* 13 (1): 40–56. https://doi.org/10.1080/0961452022000037973.

Simpson, Bob. 2004a. "Acting Ethically, Responding Culturally: Framing the New Reproductive and Genetic Technologies in Sri Lanka." *Asia Pacific Journal of Anthropology* 5 (3): 227–43. https://doi.org/10.1080/1444221042000299574.

——. 2004b, ed. *Between Macro-Ethics and Micro-Realities: What Might an Anthropology of Bioethics Look Like.* London: Wellcome Trust.

——. 2004c. "Impossible Gifts: Bodies, Buddhism and Bioethics in Contemporary Sri Lanka." *Journal of the Royal Anthropological Institute* 10 (4): 839–59. https://doi.org/10.1111/j.1467-9655.2004.00214.x.

——. 2004d. *Localising a Brave New World: New Reproductive Technologies and the Politics of Fertility in Contemporary Sri Lanka.* Edited by M. Unnithan-Kumar. *Reproductive Agency, Medicine and the State.* Oxford: Berghahn Books.

——. 2005. "Response to Athula Sumathipala and Sisira Siribaddana, 'Revisiting "Freely Given Informed Consent" in Relation to the Developing World: The Role of an Ombudsman' (AJOB 4:3)." *American Journal of Bioethics* 5 (1) W24–26. https://doi.org/10.1080/15265160590944148.

——. 2006. "'You Don't Do Fieldwork, Fieldwork Does You': Between Subjectivation and Objectivation in Anthropological Fieldwork." In *The SAGE Handbook of Fieldwork*, edited by Dick Hobbes and Richard Wright, 125–37. London: Sage.

——. 2007a. "Negotiating the Therapeutic Gap: Prenatal Diagnostics and Termination of Pregnancy in Sri Lanka." *Journal of Bioethical Inquiry* 4 (3): 207–15. http://link.springer.com/article/10.1007/s11673-007-9070-5.

——. 2007b. "On Parrots and Thorns: Sri Lankan Perspective on Genetics, Science and Personhood." *Health Care Analysis* 15 (1): 41–49. https://doi.org/10.1007/s10728-006 -0036-2.

——. 2011. "Ethical Moments: Future Directions for Ethical Review and Ethnography." *Journal of the Royal Anthropological Institute* 17 (2): 377–93. https://doi.org/10.1111 /j.1467-9655.2011.01685.x.

——. 2012. "Building Capacity: Sri Lankan Perspectives on Research, Ethics and Accountability." In *Collaborators Collaborating: Counterparts in Anthropological Knowledge and International Research Collaborations*, edited by Monica Konrad, 147–64. New York: Berghahn Books.

——. 2018. "A 'We' Problem for Bioethics and the Social Sciences: A Response to Barbara Prainsack." *Science, Technology, and Human Values* 43 (1): 45–55. https://doi.org /10.1177/0162243917735899.

Simpson, Bob, Rekha Khatri, Deapica Ravindran, and Tharindi Udalagama. 2015. "Pharmaceuticalisation and Ethical Review in South Asia: Issues of Scope and Authority for Practitioners and Policy Makers." *Social Science and Medicine* 131 (April): 247–54. https://doi.org/10.1016/j.socscimed.2014.03.016.

Simpson, E. 2014. *The Political Biography of an Earthquake: Aftermath and Amnesia in Gujarat, India*. London: Hurst.

——. 2016. "Is Anthropology Legal? Earthquake, Blitzkrieg, and Ethical Futures." *Focaal: Journal of Global and Historical Anthropology* 74 (1): 113–28. https://doi.org/10 .3167/fcl.2016.740109.

Singh, Jerome A., and Edward J. Mills. 2005. "The Abandoned Trials of Pre-Exposure Prophylaxis for HIV: What Went Wrong?" *PLoS Medicine* 2 (9): e234. https://doi.org /10.1371/journal.pmed.0020234.

Siriwardhana, Chesmal, Suwin Hewage, Ruwan Deshabandu, Sisira Siribaddana, and Athula Sumathipala. 2012. "Psychosocial and Ethical Response to Disasters: A SWOT Analysis of Post-Tsunami Disaster Management in Sri Lanka." *Asian Bioethics Review* 4 (3): 171–82. https://doi.org/10.1353/asb.2012.0027.

Siriwardhana, Chesmal, and K. Wickramage. 2014. "Conflict, Forced Displacement and Health in Sri Lanka: A Review of the Research Landscape." *Conflict and Health* 8: 22. https://doi.org/10.1186/1752-1505-8-22.

Sismondo, S. 2009. "Ghosts in the Machine: Publication Planning in the Medical Sciences." *Social Studies of Science* 39 (2): 171–98. https://doi.org/10.1177/0306312708101047.

Spencer, Jonathan. 1990. "Collective Violence and Everyday Practice in Sri Lanka." *Modern Asian Studies* 24 (3): 603–23. https://doi.org/10.1017/S0026749X00010489.

Stark, Laura. 2011. *Behind Closed Doors: IRBs and the Making of Ethical Research*. Vol. 1. Chicago: University of Chicago Press.

Stengers, Isabelle. 2010. *Cosmopolitics I*. Minneapolis: University of Minnesota Press.

Stevens, Phillips. 2004. "Diseases of Poverty and the 90/10 Gap." London: International Policy Network. http://www.who.int/intellectualproperty/submissions/International PolicyNetwork.pdf.

Strathern, Marilyn. 2000. "The Tyranny of Transparency." *British Educational Research Journal* 26 (3): 309–21. https://doi.org/10.1080/713651562.

———. 2005. *Partial Connections.* Walnut Creek, CA: Altamira Press.

———. 2011. "Can One Rely on Knowledge?" In *Evidence, Ethos and Experiment: The Anthropology and History of Medical Research in Africa,* edited by P. Wenzel Geissler and Catherine Molyneux, 57–76. New York: Berghahn Books.

———. 2012. "Currencies of Collaboration." In *Collaborators Collaborating: Counterparts in Anthropological Knowledge and International Research Collaborations,* edited by Monica Konrad, 109–25. New York: Berghahn Books.

Sumathipala, Athula. 2006. "Bioethics in Sri Lanka." *Eastern Mediterranean Health Journal* 12 (Suppl. 1): 61–67. http://www.ird.lk/wp-content/uploads/2015/03/Bioethics-in -Sri-Lanka.pdf.

Sumathipala, Athula, Aamir Jafarey, Leonardo D. De Castro, Aasim Ahmad, Darryl Macer, Sandya Srinivasan, Nandini Kumar, et al. 2010. "Ethical Issues in Post-Disaster Clinical Interventions and Research: A Developing World Perspective. Key Findings from a Drafting and Consensus Generation Meeting of the Working Group on Disaster Research and Ethics (WGDRE) 2007." *Asian Bioethics Review* 2 (2): 124–42. https://muse.jhu.edu/article/416387.

Sumathipala, Athula, and Sisira Siribaddana. 2003. *Research Ethics from a Developing World Perspective.* Colombo, Sri Lanka: Vijitha Yapa.

———. 2004. "Revisiting 'Freely Given Informed Consent' in Relation to the Developing World: Role of an Ombudsman." *American Journal of Bioethics* 4 (3): W1–7. https:// doi.org/10.1080/15265160490505498.

Sumathipala, Athula, Sisira Siribaddana, Suwin Hewage, Manura Lekamwattage, Manjula Athukorale, Chesmal Siriwardhana, Kumudu Munasinghe, et al. 2010. "Understanding of Research: A Sri Lankan Perspective." *BMC Medical Ethics* 11 (1): 7. https:// doi.org/10.1186/1472-6939-11-7.

Sumathipala, Athula, Sisira Siribaddana, Suwin Hewage, Manura Lekamwattage, Manjula Athukorale, Chesmal Siriwardhana, Joanna Murray, et al. 2008. "Informed Consent in Sri Lanka: A Survey among Ethics Committee Members." *BMC Medical Ethics* 9 (1): 10. https://doi.org/10.1186/1472-6939-9-10.

Sumathipala, Athula, Sisira Siribaddana, and Vikram Patel. 2004. "Under-Representation of Developing Countries in the Research Literature: Ethical Issues Arising from a Survey of Five Leading Medical Journals." *BMC Medical Ethics* 5 (1): E5. https://doi.org /10.1186/1472-6939-5-5.

Sumathipala, Athula, Sisira Siribaddana, Sudath Samaraweera, and D. A. R. K. Dayaratne. 2003. "Capacity Building through Multi-Disciplinary Research: A Report from Sri Lanka." *British Journal of Psychiatry* 183 (5): 457–58. https://doi.org/10.1192 /bjp.183.5.457.

Sunder Rajan, Kaushik. 2005. "Subjects of Speculation: Emergent Life Sciences and Market Logics in the United States and India." *American Anthropologist* 107 (1): 19–30. https://doi.org/10.1525/aa.2005.107.1.019.

———. 2006. *Biocapital: The Constitution of Postgenomic Life.* Durham, NC: Duke University Press.

Suryanarayanan, S., and D. L. Kleinman. 2013. "Be(e)coming Experts: The Controversy over Insecticides in the Honey Bee Colony Collapse Disorder." *Social Studies of Science* 43 (2): 215–40. https://doi.org/10.1177/0306312712466186.

Taussig, Karen-Sue, Klaus Hoeyer, and Stefan Helmreich. 2013. "The Anthropology of Potentiality in Biomedicine." *Current Anthropology* 54 (Suppl. 7): S3–14. https://doi .org/10.1086/671401.

Ten Have, H., and B. Gordijn. 2011. "Travelling Bioethics." *Medicine, Health Care and Philosophy* 14 (1): 1–3. https://doi.org/10.1007/s11019-010-9300-1.

Thagard, Paul. 2006. "How to Collaborate: Procedural Knowledge in the Cooperative Development of Science." *Southern Journal of Philosophy* 44 (Suppl. 1): 177–96. https:// doi.org/10.1111/j.2041-6962.2006.tb00038.x.

Thalagala, N. 2011. "Suicide Trends in Sri Lanka 1880–2006; Social, Demographic and Geographical Variations." *Journal of the College of Community Physicians of Sri Lanka* 14 (1): 24–32. https://doi.org/10.4038/jccpsl.v14i1.2945.

Thoradeniya, Darshi N. Forthcoming. "Sri Lanka as a Laboratory for Pill Trials in South Asia (1950–1980)." *Medical History*.

Ticktin, M. 2006. "Where Ethics and Politics Meet: The Violence of Humanitarianism in France." *American Ethnologist* 33 (1): 33–49. http://www.jstor.org/stable/3805315.

Timmermans, Stefan. 2010. "The Joy of Science: Finding Success in a Failed" Randomized Clinical Trial." *Science, Technology and Human Values* 36 (4): 549–72. https://doi .org/10.1177/0162243910366155.

Timmermans, Stefan, and Marc Berg. 2003. *The Gold Standard: The Challenge of Evidence-Based Medicine and Standardization in Health Care.* Philadelphia: Temple University Press.

Trawick, M. 1990. *Notes on Love in a Tamil Family.* Berkeley: University of California Press.

Tsing, Anna L. 2004. *Friction: An Ethnography of Global Connection.* Princeton, NJ: New Jersey: Princeton University Press.

Turner, L. 2003. "Bioethics in a Multicultural World: Medicine and Morality in Pluralistic Settings." *Health Care Analysis* 11 (2): 99–117. https://doi.org/10.1023 /A:1025620211852.

Ukpong, Morenike, and Kris Peterson, eds. 2009. "Oral Tenofovir Controversy II: Voices from the Field. A Series of Reports of the Oral Tenofovir Trials from the Perspectives of Active Community Voices Engaged in the Field in Cambodia, Cameroon, Nigeria, Thailand and Malawi." Falomo, Lagos, Nigeria: New HIV Vaccines and Microbicides Society (NHVMAS). http://www.nhvmas-ng.org/publication/TDF2.pdf.

United Nations Education, Scientific and Cultural Organisation (UNESCO). 2005. "Universal Declaration on Bioethics and Human Rights." http://www.unesco.org /education/information/50y/nfsunesco/doc/hum-rights.htm.

Uragoda, C. G. 1987. *A History of Medicine in Sri Lanka.* Colombo, Sri Lanka: Sri Lankan Medical Association. http://pgimrepository.cmb.ac.lk:8180/handle/123456789/6906.

Valdez-Martinez, E., B. Turnbull, J. Garduno-Espinosa, and J. Porter. 2006. "Descriptive Ethics: A Qualitative Study of Local Research Ethics Committees in Mexico." *Developing World Bioethics* 6 (2): 95–105. https://doi.org/10.1111/j.1471-8847.2006.00144.x.

Vidanapathirana, U. 2007. "Emerging Income Inequality and the Widening Economic Divide: The Case of Sri Lanka." Paper presented at IDEAs Conference on Policy Perspectives on Growth, Economic Structures and Poverty Reduction at Tsinghua University, Beijing, 7–9 June.

Wagner, Caroline S. 2008. *The New Invisible College: Science for Development.* Washington, DC: Brookings Institution.

Wahlberg, Ayo, Christoph Rehmann-Sutter, Margaret Sleeboom-Faulkner, Guangxiu Lu, Ole Döring, Yali Cong, Alicja Laska-Formejster, et al. 2013. "From Global Bioethics to Ethical Governance of Biomedical Research Collaborations." *Social Science and Medicine* 98 (December): 293–300. https://doi.org/10.1016/j.socscimed.2013.03.041.

Weerasuriya, N., and Saroj Jayasinghe. 2005. "A Preliminary Study of the Hospital-Admitted Older Patients in a Sri Lankan Tertiary Care Hospital." *Ceylon Medical Journal* 50 (1): 18–19. http://imsear.li.mahidol.ac.th/handle/123456789/48553.

Westbrook, David A. 2009. *Navigators of the Contemporary: Why Ethnography Matters.* Chicago: University of Chicago Press.

White, Louise. 2011. "Differences in Medicine, Differences in Ethics: Or, When Is It Research and When Is It Kidnapping or Is That Even the Right Question?" In *Evidence, Ethos and Experiment: The Anthropology and History of Medical Research in Africa*, edited by P. Wenzel Geissler and Sassy Molyneux, 445–63. New York: Berghahn Books.

Whyte, Susan Reynolds. 2011. "Writing Knowledge and Acknowledgement: Possibilities in Medical Research." In *Evidence, Ethos and Experiment: The Anthropology and History of Medical Research in Africa*, edited by P. Wenzel Geissler and Sassy Molyneux, 29–56. New York: Berghahn Books.

Wickramasinghe, Nira. 2014. *Sri Lanka in the Modern Age: A History.* Oxford: Oxford University Press. http://ier.sagepub.com/content/47/2/269.

Wickrematunge, Raisa. 2012. "Controversy over Clinical Drug Trials." *Sunday Leader*, March 4. http://www.thesundayleader.lk/2012/03/04/controversy-over-clinical-drug-trials/.

Widger, Tom. 2012. "Suffering, Frustration, and Anger: Class, Gender and History in Sri Lankan Suicide Stories." *Culture, Medicine and Psychiatry* 36 (2): 225–44. https://doi.org/10.1007/s11013-012-9250-6.

Widger, Tom, and S. Kabir. n.d. "An Appropriate Sacrifice: Perfections of Generosity and the Politics of Elders Charity in Sri Lanka." Unpublished manuscript.

Wilks, Martin F, Ravindra Fernando, P. L. Ariyananda, Michael Eddleston, David J. Berry, John A. Tomenson, Nicholas A. Buckley, Shaluka Jayamanne, David Gunnell, and Andrew Dawson. 2008. "Improvement in Survival after Paraquat Ingestion Following Introduction of a New Formulation in Sri Lanka." *PLoS Medicine* 5 (2): 0250–59. https://doi.org/10.1371/journal.pmed.0050049.

Williams, Simon J., Paul Martin, and Jonathan Gabe. 2011. "The Pharmaceuticalisation of Society? A Framework for Analysis." *Sociology of Health and Illness* 33 (5): 710–25. https://doi.org/10.1111/j.1467-9566.2011.01320.x.

World Health Organization (WHO). 1995. "Guidelines for Good Clinical Practice (GCP) for Trials on Pharmaceutical Products." WHO Technical Report Series. Geneva: World Health Organization. http://apps.who.int/medicinedocs/collect/medicinedocs/pdf/whozip13e/whozip13e.pdf.

World Medical Association (WMA). 2013. "Declaration of Helsinki: Ethical Principles for Medical Research Involving Human Subjects." *JAMA* 310 (20): 2191–94. https://doi.org/10.1001/jama.2013.281053.

Wray, K. B. 2002. "The Epistemic Significance of Collaborative Research." *Philosophy of Science* 69 (1): 150–68. https://doi.org/10.1086/338946.

Yarrow, Thomas, and Soumhya Venkatesan. 2012. "Anthropology and Development: Critical Framings." In *Differentiating Development: Beyond an Anthropology of Critique*, edited by Thomas Yarrow and Soumhya Venkatesan, 1–20. Oxford: Berghahn Books.

Yuval, R., and D. A. Halon. 2000. "Patient Comprehension and Reaction to Participating in a Double-Blind Randomized Clinical Trial (ISIS-4) in Acute Myocardial Infarction." *Archives of Internal Medicine* 160: 1142–46. https://doi.org/10.1001/archinte.160.8.1142.

Zabusky, S. E. 2000. "Boundaries at Work: Discourses and Practices of Belonging in the European Space Agency." In *An Anthropology of the European Union: Building, Imaging and Experiencing the New Europe*, edited by I. Bellier and T. M. Wilson, 179–200. Oxford: Berghahn Books.

Zong, Z. 2008. "Should Post-Trial Provision of Beneficial Experimental Interventions Be Mandatory in Developing Countries?" *Journal of Medical Ethics* 34: 188–92. https://doi.org/10.1136/jme.2006.018754.

Zvonareva, Olga, Natalia Kutishenko, Evgeny Kulikov, and Sergey Martsevich. 2015. "Risks and Benefits of Trial Participation: A Qualitative Study of Participants' Perspectives in Russia." *Clinical Trials* 12 (6): 646–53. https://doi.org/10.1177/1740774515589592.

Index

Lightning Source UK Ltd.
Milton Keynes UK
UKHW010624171221
395726UK00002B/74